OSTEOPATHY

A practising osteopathic practiti͏   ͏͏cept of
osteopathy, reviews modern dev͏   ͏͏ and shows clearly
what its potentials are for the alleviation of a wide range of
health problems.

By the same author:
ABOUT LAETRILE
ACUPUNCTURE TREATMENT OF PAIN
AN END TO CANCER?
INSTANT PAIN CONTROL
NEURO-MUSCULAR TECHNIQUE

OSTEOPATHY

A Complete Health-care System

by
Leon Chaitow
N.D., D.O., M.B.N.O.A.

Series Editor
George T. Lewith
M.A., M.R.C.G.P., M.R.C.P.

THORSONS PUBLISHERS LIMITED
Wellingborough, Northamptonshire

First published 1982

British Library Cataloguing in Publication Data

Chaitow, Leon
  Osteopathy
  1. Osteopathy
  I. Title
  615.5'33   RZ341

  ISBN 0-7225-0782-8
  ISBN 0-7225-0745-3 Pbk

Printed and bound in Great Britain

Acknowledgements

The most far reaching scientific research into physiological function related to osteopathy has been carried out over the past thirty-five years by Professor Irvin M. Korr Ph.D. He has generously consented to my quoting from his published papers, and I wish to acknowledge this with thanks.

My thanks also go to the distinguished editor of the Journal of the American Osteopathic Association, George W. Northup D.O., for granting permission to quote from those of Professor Korr's works that first appeared in that excellent publication.

I wish to thank Professor Michael Patterson Ph.D. of the College of Osteopathic Medicine, Ohio State University, for his kind permission to quote from his writings. Finally, my thanks go to the memory of Andrew Taylor Still for discovering the truths which live on in osteopathy today.

For Alkmini and Sasha

Contents

Foreword

Spinal manipulation has its origins in the ancient art of bone-setting. Osteopathy uses refined and sophisticated manipulative therapy based on the teachings of an American, Dr Andrew Taylor Still. It embraces the idea of 'whole person' medicine and looks upon the system of muscles, bones and joints — particularly the spine — as reflecting the body's diseases, and also as being partially responsible for initiating disease processes. At first it is difficult to conceive of the mechanism in which a minor spinal problem will initiate disease in the heart or lungs. However, it is apparent from the evidence provided that this can occur.

Leon Chaitow has condensed and explained many of the complex and difficult concepts of osteopathy in a clear and understandable manner. There is obviously a great deal of further research required in this field before the case for osteopathy is proven, but it is undoubtedly a therapy that is effective for many people and therefore must be worthy of further serious and detailed consideration.

The history of osteopathy has not always been smooth, many people have thought it little more than quackery. This concise and objective summary of the subject will allow the reader to make up his own mind and decide for himself whether osteopathy has anything to offer as a therapy.

GEORGE LEWITH M.A., M.R.C.G.P., M.R.C.P.
Southampton

Introduction

Osteopathy, having entered its second century of existence as a means of healing, is still much misunderstood, and the aim of this book is to dispel many popular misconceptions and to explain just what it is all about.

Osteopathy is a system of healing which is practised throughout the world, and in America and Great Britain in particular it has achieved a wide public acceptance of its value. An ever-increasing number of medical and paramedical practitioners are studying its methods or are recommending its use, but many still have a narrow view of osteopathy's range of application. This book is aimed at widening that view.

Whilst justifiable attention is focused on nutrition and emotional factors in restoring health, the structural element has frequently been ignored. Whether a patient is concerned with relatively simple mechanical dysfunction, such as might occur in backache or a stiff neck, or whether the problem is of a more complex nature, such as migraine or asthma, there is a need for him to know just how manipulation of the structure of the body might be able to help.

The osteopath examines the patient with one basic aim in mind; to find and correct that which is structurally incorrect, and to thus restore normal function wherever possible. There are many methods, and many techniques — some subtle and some forceful — used by osteopaths in achieving this aim, and relatively recently developments such as cranial manipulation, especially for use on infants injured in childbirth, has opened new vistas for the modern osteopath.

Properly applied, osteopathic manipulation will have no side-effects. It is an energy saving system in that there is no expensive energy-consuming equipment involved, only the hands of the practitioner, and it is time saving since the majority of musculo-skeletal conditions respond rapidly to osteopathic treatment.

1. What is Osteopathy?

If you have ever had an aching back, stiff neck, tennis elbow, 'gammy' knee or some such affliction of the body, then the chances are that you have sought the help of, or have been advised by someone to go to, an osteopath for relief. If, however, you have, or have had, a more serious health problem such as asthma, migraine headaches, angina pains, digestive disturbances (to name but a few examples), then it has probably not occurred to you that the condition might have some of its origins in a dysfunction of some mechanical component of the body, the musculo-skeletal system. You would, therefore, probably not have taken such a problem to an osteopath practitioner. Surprising as it may seem, many such 'illnesses' are often the end result of biomechanical changes in the structure of the body which are amenable to osteopathic treatment. This theme will be elaborated on in later chapters, and some of the fascinating research that has been done in a wide range of health problems will be detailed. At this stage, the idea of osteopathy offering help to conditions other than the more obvious aches and pains may seem a strange one. In order to understand the concept of osteopathy, and what its real potentials are, it is necessary to examine its roots and subsequent development.

Osteopathy is a system of health care which recognizes that the self-healing, self-regulating ability of the body is dependent upon a number of factors, including favourable environmental conditions (internal and external), adequate nutrition and normal structural integrity. It utilizes generally accepted methods of diagnosis, as well as certain specialised ones developed to facilitate accurate structural assessment. It places special emphasis upon the importance of body mechanics, and uses manipulative techniques to detect and correct, faulty structure and function.

In many people's minds, especially in the U.K., osteopathy is equated mainly with the treatment of spinal and other joint pains and problems. This limited care concept is largely an historical accident. As indicated above, the osteopathic profession sees itself as being relevant to a wide range of health problems, and not simply limited to the treatment of musculo-

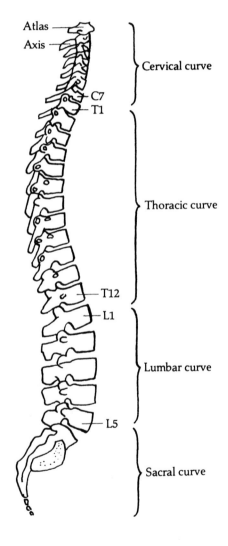

Side view of a normal spine showing the natural curves.

skeletal derangements. Since the turn of the century, when the first American-trained osteopaths established themselves in practice in the U.K., they have filled a gap that existed (and to a large extent still exists) in medical practice. Doctors tended to regard musculo-skeletal problems as relatively unimportant, and manipulation as, at best, an unknown quantity and, at worst, valueless.

In the U.S.A., the gradual evolution of osteopathy has been towards its original goal of providing a complete health-care system, dealing with all of man's ailments, and utilizing all those accepted therapeutic methods which coincide with its belief in the necessity for treating the patient as a whole, rather than simply treating symptoms. This concept of treating the 'whole' man deserves closer scrutiny. Disease may be stated to be the result of a disparity between the capacities, resources and responses of the individual, and the demands and circumstances made by his life. Disease can be seen to be a phase in the natural history of the individual, whose unique nature responds to his own particular environment. The individual's inheritance, capacities, resources and demands, and, therefore, his adaptations and responses, are unique to him. Illness, the level of health, predispositions, resistance, responses, adaptations etc. to all the elements of his environment, are a culmination of an individual's life, up to that point. The apparent similarities between diseases in different individuals, and the ability to classify diseases, are testimony to the fact that the body can respond in only a limited number of ways to an infinite variety of events and factors. The patient's illness should, therefore, not be seen to be a disease, or aberration, of an organ or process alone, but as part of an illness in his total being. The patient with angina is not ill because of his angina, but has angina because he is ill. It is consideration of the whole picture of the patient's uniqueness, and his relationship with all his complex environmental factors, that provide the background for the total health care that osteopathy seeks to offer. This, of course, includes consideration of the largest body system, the musculo-skeletal system. The methods of care also include its own distinctive approach to the normalizing of musculo-skeletal dysfunction, osteopathic manipulative therapy (O.M.T.).

It is not possible to separate osteopathic practice from the theories that produced it. Osteopathy is not just a mechanistic approach to disease but a sincere and effective system which attempts to remove the causes of ill-health and seeks to reinforce the basic curative force which lies within the body itself. This belief was originally expressed over a hundred years ago by Andrew Taylor Still, the originator of Osteopathy, whose life and work will be considered in the next chapter. The concept of many of the causes, and therefore of the remedies, lying within the body itself, has a long history. For as long as man has existed on earth, disease and injury have existed with him.

Treatment of disease was, in prehistory, asssigned to practitioners of one or another healing method. The cause of disease was ascribed, by many, to outside forces which were thought to enter the body of the sufferer. Treatment in such a case was aimed at driving out such evil or morbid influences. Other practitioners blamed aberrations within the body, or soul, of the victim, for the disease process, and treatment was then designed to normalize the causative disturbances. These two divergent philosophies, the outside or inside cause, existed side by side for centuries.

In the fourth century B.C. a rational system of healing was introduced by the great Greek physician Hippocrates. He taught that illness was often caused by quite simple things, such as eating the wrong food or by living in unhygienic conditions. He therefore recognized that the apparent causes of disease could originate from external or internal factors. However, he believed also that the body itself, through the healing efforts of its own nature, was the means of recovery. 'It is our natures that are the physicians of our diseases'.

He stressed that the physician should assist the ability of the body to overcome disease by removing causative factors, and by encouraging the healing effort, but never to meddle with, or hinder nature's attempt towards recovery. Thus the school of thought that followed Hippocrates' teaching emphasized the study of health of man as a whole integrated unit; relating the whole man to his environment. Within that framework the causes of ill health were to be found.

Other schools of thought, however, continued to focus attention on the disease process itself, as an entity, largely ignoring the patient. The history of medicine ever since has been highlighted by proponents of one or other of these schools of thought. Through the ages we find the theoretical battle raging which is more important, the diseased or the disease? It is true to say that the Hippocratic concept has been more honoured, but the rival philosophy has been more practised.

Osteopathic theory and practice are firmly in line with the concepts of Hippocrates. The patient is considered and treated as a whole. Founded as it was in this tradition, osteopathy is patient orientated rather than disease orientated. It has utilized structural diagnosis and manipulative therapy as part of its philosophy and practice, and therefore as part of total patient care, not confining it to painful conditions of the musculo-skeletal system alone.

In essence the original concept of osteopathy held that:

1. Within the human body there exists a constant tendency towards health. If this capacity is recognized, and if treatment takes its relevance into account, then the prevention and normalization of disease processes is enhanced.

2. The structure of the body is reciprocally related to its function. By this it is meant that any change in structure will alter some aspect of function and, conversely, any alteration in function will result in structural changes.

3. Health is the primary area to be studied in attempting to understand disease.

4. The musculo-skeletal system, which incorporates the bones, ligaments, muscles, fascia etc. forms a structure which, when disordered, may affect the function of other parts and systems of the body. This might be the result of irritation or abnormal response of the nerve and/or blood supply to these other organs or parts.

5. The body is subject to mechanical disorder and is therefore capable of mechanical correction.

Discussion of these concepts will be found in the chapter dealing with osteopathic theory.

There is a growing awareness of the value to general health of an integrated, mechanically sound, musculo-skeletal system. The scientific rationale for this becomes clearer with research. Clinically, however, osteopaths have long realized the positive effects of manipulative therapy on health. It is necessary to keep in mind two essentially different roles filled by Osteopathic practitioners in their work. One is that of providing limited care to patients with joint pains and strains. The other is the total health-care of patients, with any of the myriad ills of mankind. There is also a further extension of osteopathic care, in areas in which no other form of healing offers much help. This is the more recent application of osteopathic principles and methods to the structures (bones, reciprocal tension membranes, fluid fluctuations etc.) of the skull, especially of infants. As will be described in the chapter on Cranial Osteopathy. These methods, when successfully applied to such problems as cerebral palsy and spasticity of the newborn, can produce results bordering on the miraculous. In its limited application (joint injuries, postural stresses etc.) osteopathy is a most effective system for the treatment of musculo-skeletal derangements.

Osteopathy Compared
Confusion exists in both public and medical minds as to the distinction between osteopathic and other forms of physical treatment. Because other systems utilize manipulative methods on their approach to the patient it is often assumed, even by apparently knowledgeable individuals, that there really is not very much difference between osteopathy and, for example, physiotherapy or chiropractic. Nothing could be further from the truth, and a brief examination of some of the other systems with which osteopathy is often confused should help to clarify the differences.

Chiropractic
Osteopathy and chiropractic differ in three main areas. These are the philosophical or theoretical aspects, the technique and the training. Osteopathy has a basic philosophical viewpoint from which have developed the specialized diagnostic and therapeutic measures, including osteopathic manipulative technique.

Chiropractic originally placed great emphasis on the idea that spinal joints, when misplaced (subluxated), could impinge upon nerves and thus cause disease elsewhere in the body. Chiropractors tended to focus attention on the spinal and pelvic structures, employing elaborate x-ray procedures in their analysis of subluxations. Treatment tended to be by specific high velocity thrust techniques, often employing a rebound effect from complex, sprung treatment couches.

Over the years chiropractic has tended to take more and more interest in joint dysfunction as related to back and neck pain rather than in the general treatment of ill health. A survey in

Australia, Canada and the U.K. indicated that 90 per cent of patients attending chiropractors do so for treatment of low back and neck pain. Chiropractic techniques have also changed over the years, to the point where many practitioners employ similar functional and leverage techniques to osteopaths. In the same way, many osteopaths have incorporated thrust techniques usually associated with chiropractic.

In the U.S.A. osteopathy has become an accepted (in law) alternative system to orthodox medicine, employing its own unique methods as well as what it considers useful from the orthodox system, in the treatment of all forms of ill health. Chiropractic is more limited in its legal position, its range of application and in its range of methods. It is certainly true to say, though, that in treatment of neck and back conditions the difference between the two systems has become blurred. The training of an osteopath in the U.S.A. takes seven years and a full licence is granted to graduates. A four year training which is undertaken to achieve a chiropractic doctorate leads to a limited licence (no surgery, drug prescription or the right to sign death certificates etc.)

Historically the two professions grew out of similar roots, but they have evolved to the point where their similarities are to be seen only in the relatively narrow areas of pain and dysfunction in the back and neck. Their differences become very apparent in their consideration of general health care.

Manipulative Therapy

This has grown out of the tradition of remedial massage and bonesetting. Whilst utilizing techniques which resemble osteopathic manipulative therapy and chiropractic, manipulative therapists regard their work as being aimed at the physical normalization of joint and muscle dysfunction, with the objective of improving mechanical function. No attempt is made to relate the methods to broader aspects of body function or ill health; indeed such ideas are actively discouraged by the leaders of this profession, which sees itself as a system subsidiary to medicine, in contrast to osteopathy which sees itself as an alternative.

Most of the work of these therapists involves massage, with manipulation only being used when considered absolutely necessary. There are no full time training facilities for such practitioners who are, as a rule, physiotherapists or masseurs drawn to these methods. Some are skillful and competent, but their narrow view as to the value and application of manipulation, together with their limited approach to bodily dysfunction, distinguishes them from the osteopathic practitioner.

Bonesetters
There are still some 'bonesetters' about, especially in remote rural areas. These are, frequently, gifted healers carrying on an unwritten tradition of learned and acquired skills which go back into prehistory.

In England, there was for many centuries a tradition of bonesetters. Many of these undoubtedly skilled practitioners had no formal medical training. In the early eighteenth century a Mrs Mapp achieved a great following and was consulted by many doctors.

In 1867 Sir James Paget, an eminent physician, warned his fellow doctors: 'Few of you are likely to practice without having a bonesetter for a rival; and if he can cure a case which you have failed to cure, his fortune will be made and yours marred.'

The fame of Herbert Barker, an unqualified bonesetter, was so great that he was eventually knighted for his services. He was hounded by orthodox medicine and all contact between Barker and doctors was forbidden on pain of expulsion from the profession; this, despite his continual stream of successful cases. In his old age Barker demonstrated his techniques to a group of orthopaedic surgeons in London, a final admission of his genius.

Manipulation, as practised by bonesetters, was a relatively simple matter of pushing or pulling restricted joints, to achieve ease of movement. Sometimes great force was used and frequently damage was caused by excessive violence. The difference between such methods and their total lack of any coherent or systematic use differentiates them from osteopathy.

Massage
Massage has a long history, but not until the nineteenth century was a systematic approach developed by P. H. Ling in Sweden. A school of medical gymnastics was founded, and this promoted the use of 'scientific' massage. Many variations exist. Some methods are remedial, being aimed at the restoration of function lost during surgery or because of enforced bed-rest (accidents, strokes etc.), or through advancing age. Other

methods are used to encourage function in birth injuries or disease-damaged (polio) patients. Massage techniques are also used in gaining general relaxation and circulatory improvements.

Osteopaths utilize specialized soft-tissue techniques which bear a superficial resemblance to massage. Both deal with the soft tissues. The osteopath is either preparing the area for subsequent manipulation or dealing reflexly with problems distant from the area being treated. The U.K. trained osteopath might use a system developed in England known as neuro-muscular technique. In the U.S.A a similar deep soft tissue method was developed by the late Ida Rolf. Both these methods have some similarities with the specialized German method of connective tissue massage (Bindesgewebsmassage) which uses deep finger and thumb strokes to achieve local and reflex effects. Rolfing aims at releasing deep tissue contractions and thus encouraging postural and structural reintegration, and psychological 'release' from emotions which are tied into muscular stress patterns. Neuro-muscular technique, rolfing and connective tissue massage are all specialized soft tissue methods, bearing little in common with what is normally thought of as massage.

Physiotherapy

In orthodox medicine the remedial gymnast and masseur of old has been replaced by the physiotherapist of today. This profession is an adjunct of the dominant medical system, and it incorporates a variety of modalities such as exercise, massage and manipulation. Traction and some forms of hydrotherapy also form part of the physiotherapist's methods. In other words, anything that can usefully be employed in treating the physical body, to enhance its function, or to minimize its dysfunction, especially as related to the muscles and joints, is incorporated into physiotherapy. There are, of course, other rehabilitative aspects and therapeutic ones (such as encouraging normality after injury or surgery, and assisting in respiratory function in asthmatics.)

In the main, however, physiotherapists deal with the vast range of rheumatic diseases with the modalities outlined. Their use of manipulation tends to be confined to a limited range of specific techniques which are applied to the neck and low back areas. The techniques employed are usually direct action ones where joints are forced through a range of motion.

Doctors of physical medicine and orthopaedic surgeons tend to limit their sphere of interest to the mechanics and pathology of the musculo-skeletal system. This is a large and vital area, but from the osteopathic viewpoint it is important, not only in itself, but because of the ramifications that dysfunction in any of its constituent parts may have on the overall economy of the body and on specific organs and functions.

As we shall see in the unfolding of the history and current practice of osteopathy, as important as manipulative methods and specialized osteopathic diagnostic methods are to the science of osteopathy, it has always been recognized that care of the 'whole' man requires the integration and use of all methods and measures which contribute to well-being. This was made clear in the charter of the first College of Osteopathy in 1892. The aim then was stated to be 'To establish a college of osteopathy, the design of which is to improve our present system of surgery, obstetrics and treatment of diseases generally, and to place the same on a more scientific and rational basis and to impart knowledge to the medical profession'. A reforming role was seen as being the essential part osteopathic medicine would play. The subsequent history and the success of the profession especially in the country of its birth, against extraordinary odds, is fascinating. Before we touch on this, however, a man of extraordinary vision deserves our attention; Andrew Taylor Still.

2. The Birth of Osteopathy

Manipulative methods as part of medical treatment are known to date back to earliest times. Hippocrates wrote of their value. Throughout medical history manual methods have been used, but almost always with a view to the correction of gross structural problems such as dislocations or spinal deformities. The methods used were empirical and often extremely forceful, with a minimum of scientific rationale to support their use. The same can be said for much of medical practice, until the end of the nineteenth century. Heroic drugging and bleeding were the methods most frequently used in order to bludgeon the body back to a semblance of health.

There have been a number of medical reformers who saw the folly of attacking the apparent disease process, or more often the symptoms of it, rather than seeking and eliminating causes. Among these were the celebrated Dutch physician Hermann Boerhaave (1669-1738), and the great English doctor and teacher, Thomas Sydenham. They stressed the vital importance, in the Hippocratic tradition, of placing the study of the patient at the heart of medicine rather than emphasizing the disease process.

Andrew Taylor Still

In a different age and out of a very different culture there emerged a man who wrestled with the same problems and who came to a practical solution. Andrew Taylor Still was born in 1828 in Jonesburgh, Virginia. His father Rev Abram Still, of the Methodist Episcopal Church, was both preacher and doctor to his flock. This was not an unusual combination at this time in frontier America. When Andrew was six the family moved to Tennesee, where he attended elementary school. Three years later the family moved again to Northern Missouri, Abram Still having been appointed as Methodist missionary in the area. There Andrew attended a typical frontier school.

During this period Andrew displayed a great interest in the natural environment. With his father's aid he studied and observed nature. He found great beauty and order in the world, marred only by the constant presence of disease and death. He was horrified by the havoc caused by the common diseases of the day, such as smallpox, cholera and meningitis. He was

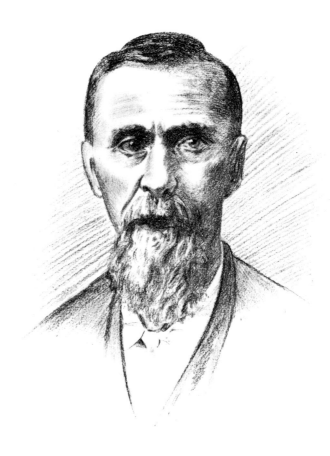

Andrew Taylor Still MD (1828-1917)
Founder of Osteopathy

sensitive to the inadequacies of current medical methods in dealing with these diseases.

When Andrew was sixteen the family moved again, this time to Kansas where his father had been appointed missionary to the Shawnee Indians. At the age of eighteen Andrew Still married. In 1857 he was elected to the Kansas legislature where he promoted the anti-slavery cause. His wife died in 1859 leaving him with three young children, and he remarried in 1860. His medical training began when he was able to help and learn from his father, and other practising doctors of medicine. At this time medical schools were few in the U.S.A. and the preceptor method of training was usual. Before the civil war he attended the College of Physicians and Surgeons in Kansas City, but before completing the course he enlisted in the army. During the civil war he served as a surgeon and rose to the rank of major.

Following the war he continued to study the nature of health and disease. He found current theory and practice inadequate and in his autobiography he states: 'I was in the practice of medicine and had been for several years. I treated my patients as other doctors did. Some of them got well, and some of them died. Others, both young and old, got sick and got well again without the assistance of the medical doctor'. He studied the human body in detail, its structure and the relationship between structure and function. He became convinced that only through an understanding of this relationship could an understanding be achieved of the malfunctions of the body, i.e. disease.

In 1864 an epidemic of meningitis struck the Missouri frontier. Thousands died, including his three children. It was his helplessness during this tragedy that drove him on in his studies. 'Not until my heart had been torn and lacerated with grief and affliction,' he wrote, 'could I fully realize the inefficacy of drugs. Some may say that I should suffer in order that good might come, but I feel that my grief came through gross ignorance on the part of the medical profession.'

This experience crystalized his dissatisfaction with the current empirical methods of medical treatment of disease. He sought a philosophy upon which to base his practice which would not vary with every new wind of doctrine or experiment, but which would have a scientific basis. This he sought at a time when modern science and methods of research were unknown, and he devoted himself to the study and analysis of all the existing knowledge available to him. On 29 August 1874 he was registered as a practising physician in Macon county, Missouri.

Shortly after this he announced the results of his years of study. He stated three fundamental principles upon which he would base his practice of medicine. These were (1) The body produces its own healing substances; (2) Health is dependent upon structural integrity; (3) Perverted structure is a fundamental cause of disease. Besides these principles he also originated a system of manipulation. Basing his philosophy of practice upon these principles he proceeded to correlate manipulative therapy with other methods, then used by doctors, such as drugs and surgery. In many instances he found that the use of manipulative methods made drugs and operations unnecessary. The concepts and theories were proved in his clinical experience. He developed the art of manipulative therapy, based on his knoweldge of human anatomy, physiology and chemistry and, above all, on his new found discovery of the vital inter-relationship between the structure of the body and its function.

An Early Case
One early case illustrates his approach at this time, and also shows the fairly primitive knowledge of the way the body functions that was prevalent at that time. Despite this obstacle Andrew Taylor Still was able to evolve and construct a theory and a practical system of therapeutics which worked then, as it does now, because it recognized and was based upon natural laws. In his autobiography he describes the case of a child with dysentery:

> I placed my hand on the back of the little fellow in the region of the lumbar and found it very warm, even hot, while the abdomen was cold. My only thought was to help . . . and little dreamed I was to make a discovery that would bless future generations. I thought it strange that the back was so hot and the belly so cold; then the neck and the back of his head were very warm and the face, forehead and nose cold. I began to reason, for I then knew very little about flux (dysentery), more than the fact that it killed old and young and was worse in warm weather. I did not know how to reason on diseases because all the authorities I had met could not get their eyes off the effects to turn them to the cause. I knew that a person had a spinal cord but little of its use. I began to work at the base of the brain and thought that by pressing and rubbing I could push some of the heat to the cold places. While doing so, I found rigid and loose places in

the child's whole spine, while the lumbar region was in a very congested condition. I worked for a few minutes on that philosophy and then told the mother to report to me the next day. She came early next morning to report that the child was well. I had seventeen severe cases of flux in a few days and cured them all without drugs.

As we shall see in later chapters, spinal manipulation is used with great benefit in many infectious diseases.

At the time Dr Still was living in Kirksville, Missouri, and his fame spread rapidly, and patients came to him from all over America. He found that by careful palpation, i.,e. examination by feeling the surface of the body, he could ascertain abnormalities, and by careful manipulation he could often restore normal function. In many cases he found that he was able to achieve beneficial results, where previously he had failed. He records success with cases of pneumonia, asthma and many acute and chronic ailments. Osteopathy, to Still, meant diagnosis followed by specific manual techniques applied spontaneously until he felt the desired changes in the tissues or joints on which he was working. He did not apply manipulation as a remedy for symptoms as such, but regarded himself as a mechanic of the living body, restoring or encouraging its natural powers of recovery.

The case of the child with dysentery illustrates how the idea evolved. Starting with the idea of moving heat from one part of the body to another he used his hands on the child's spine, felt abnormalities and proceeded to normalize these, with good effect. By trial and error he found that similar abnormal structural changes existed in many conditions and from these simple beginnings grew a new science.

The facts have not changed, such abnormalities are still to be found in most spines. We do, however, have more of an idea as to what the physiological and pathological implications of these areas are. They used to be called osteopathic lesions, and a great deal of vitriolic, not to say hysterical, attacks on the very idea of their existence, have been made by medical writers. The current osteopathic terminology labels these 'lesions' as 'areas of somatic dysfunction', and later we shall examine in more detail their significance.

Still's gifts as a skilled manipulator and healer are well documented. There was a celebrated case in which he reduced a dislocated elbow in minutes after four physicians had failed, even with the patient under anaesthesia. His contribution to the healing art was to offer an alternative to the heavy drugging of orthodox medicine of that time. He also conceived the basic theories of his new approach and developed and originated the manipulative skills without any outside aid. A man of brilliance and dedication, he stubbornly persisted in his work, despite enormous opposition from the medical establishment.

In considering his contribution, it is as well to realize that medical knowledge as we know it today was in its infancy. Antiseptic surgery was only just being introduced by Lister against conservative opposition. It was another twenty years before radiography was introduced, and the germ theory of Pasteur had only been established some ten years previously. It was in this dark age that Still worked out a practical system of structural therapeutics that has never been invalidated by later discoveries. Still emphasized the importance of the musculo-skeletal system as a major factor in disease processes; he recognized the body structure as an important source of derangement. It was therefore also a major avenue for the application of therapy designed to assist natural defences and to repair and restore physiological adaptive functions. The result of this view is to distinguish the patient from his ailment and to recognize finally that only by understanding the attributes of health can the disease process be studied and corrected.

In order to cope with the demands of some of his fellow doctors, Still trained them in his theories and techniques. This led ultimately to the founding of the first College of Osteopathy in Kirksville, in 1892. He based his school upon the fundamental principles of the osteopathic concept and included in its teachings all avaliable methods which were useful in the care of the sick. Sixteen men and three women graduated from this first Osteopathic College in 1894. From that small beginning the growth of the profession has, against great odds, been staggering. Today there are twelve osteopathic schools in the U.S.A. Some are part of major university campuses, and between them they graduate some one thousand new osteopaths annually, after seven years of training, which includes a full orthodox medical training, as well as the specialized osteopathic theories and methods.

Graduates enjoy all the rights and privileges enjoyed by graduates of medical schools. But, as we shall see in the following chapter, this position is not the case in other countries where osteopathy has yet to realize its true potential. Dr Still was an eccentric individualist who lived through a storm of abuse from the medical fraternity to the age of 89. When 'the old Doctor' died in 1917 there were more than five thousand osteopathic physicians practising in the U.S.A.

3. Development to the Present Day

From its small beginnings in the last years of the nineteenth century to the present time there has been a dynamic growth in osteopathy in all its spheres — education, research and practice. In the U.S.A there are in the region of 20,000 fully licenced osteopathic physicians currently in practice. Their training is in all respects equal to that received by medical students in terms of content, standards and requirements.

The emphasis in the osteopathic colleges has, over the years, been towards producing osteopathic practitioners who could practise comprehensive medicine, using orthodox methods as well as the unique osteopathic approach. This has tended to result in a number of osteopathic physicians becoming indistinguishable from orthodox doctors, and many have found it easier to practise 'straight' medicine rather than to employ the methods uniquely associated with osteopathy.

As a result of this trend a group of practitioners dedicated to the preservation and dissemination of the essential fundamentals of osteopathy formed, in 1937, the Academy of Applied Osteopathy. This organization, through its efforts, has been responsible for a resurgence of interest amongst the new generations of practitioners in the methods and philosophy of the origional osteopathic pioneers. The Year Books of the Academy provide a treasure-house of information and inspiration for the profession.

It should not be thought, though, that the osteopathic profession has been slavishly tied to the pronouncements of Dr Still. Indeed, as early as 1918, Dr Michael Lane D.O. wrote 'Many osteopaths, while revering the founder of the new system, have seemed to feel that because Still was right in his grand principles of disease and its therapy, that therefore he should not have been wrong in anything he said about the body and its work in health and disease. But such osteopaths are short-sighted and unwise. If Dr Still had been right in all his theories he would not have not been human.'

In the U.K., where osteopathy has had a very different history from that in the U.S.A., writers and teachers have tried to hold on to the esentials of Still's teaching whilst also being aware of his shortcomings. In 1954 the eminent British osteopath, S. Webster-Jones, describing in a lecture the case of the child with dysentery who Still had treated, said: 'It would be only too easy to ridicule Still's approach to this case, and his idea of moving heat from one part of the body to another. Discredit Still's ideas on physiology, diet, medical diagnosis, as you will, actually they led him back to his patient as a whole, to seek in his body the cause of his illness and to try to remove it. They led him away from that overstudy of local pathology and preoccupation with local and systemic diseases that has led to over-specialization in orthodox medicine, which has had the effect that the patient is often forgotten in the study of disease.'

Osteopathic Colleges in the U.S.A.

In the U.S.A. all states licence graduates of the twelve Colleges, and they are at liberty to practise unlimited medicine after seven years training. The twelve colleges are:

Chicago College of Osteopathic Medicine.
College of Osteopathic Medicine and Surgery, Des Moines, Iowa.
Kansas City College of Osteopathic Medicine.
Kirksville College of Osteopathic Medicine.
Michigan State Univeristy College of Osteopathic Medicine.
Ohio University College of Osteopathic Medicine.
Oklahoma College of Osteopathic Medicine and Surgery.
Philadelphia College of Osteopathic Medicine.
Texas College of Osteopathic Medicine.
West Virginia School of Osteopathic Medicine.
New York College of Osteopathic Medicine.
New Jersey School of Osteopathic Medicine.

New colleges are in the process of development in Maine and California. As the names indicate, there are a number of osteopathic colleges which are part of major University campuses. As also indicated, many teach surgery as an integral part of Osteopathic training.

There are, in the U.S.A., a variety of speciality groups including Anaesthesiology, General Practice, Internal Medicine, Neurology and Psychiatry, Nuclear Medicine, Obstetrics and Gynaecology, Ophthaemology and Otorhinolaryngology, Pathology, Paediatrics, Proctology, Radiology, Rehabilitation Medicine, Surgery etc. In all these specialist fields there are skilled physicians approaching their individual areas of disease or dysfunction from an osteopathic viewpoint. The growth in numbers of practitioners and colleges has been paralled by the development of osteopathic hospitals, of which there are hundreds in the U.S.A.

With more and more graduates, with the highest academic qualifications, and the constant voice of the Academy of Applied Osteopathy to remind them of their unique heritage, the 'Old doctor's' proteges would seem to have established themselves in the country of osteopathy's birth.

The Situation in the U.K.
In the U.K. osteopaths practise under common law. There is no legislation governing the right to practise or the scope of practise. Anyone with or without training may establish a practise and style themselves as an osteopath and use the initials D.O. (which in the U.K. stand for Diploma of Osteopathy). There are three colleges offering four year courses (full time) in osteopathy in the U.K. No surgery or pharmacology are taught as subjects for students in the U.K. (where a more limited approach to the health problems of the patient exists than in the U.S.A.).

The British colleges are (in order of seniority):

The British School of Osteopathy, whose graduates style themselves 'Registered Osteopaths' and use the initials M.R.O.

The British College of Osteopathy and Naturopathy, whose graduates style themselves 'Registered Naturopaths and Osteopaths' and use the initials M.B.N.O.A.

Ecole Européene d'Osteopathie, whose graduates style themselves 'Members of the Society of Osteopaths' and use the initials M.S.O.

Apart from these colleges, all of which attract discretionary grants from local authorities, there are a number of colleges and schools, offering part-time and correspondence courses. There is also The London School of Osteopathy which offers a one year post graduate course to qualified medical practitioners.

The rivalry, and lack of co-operation, between the various osteopathic groups in the U.K. until fairly recently would be laughable were it not so sad. Of the estimated three thousand practising osteopaths in the U.K., no more than 600 are graduates of full-time colleges. The remainder may have had some or no training, and whilst some of these practitioners are skillful, they patently do not have the background knowledge of anatomy and physiology possessed by the more adequately trained practitioners.

A further area of discord results from the strict code of ethics insisted upon by the associations governing the graduates of the full time colleges. Among the rules affecting these practitioners is a prohibition on advertising in any shape or form. The less well qualified osteopaths, who are not elligible for membership of the three main organizations (whose members are identified by the letters M.R.O., M.B.N.O.A., or M.S.O.) can, and do, advertise. The College of Osteopaths, which offers a five-year part-time training also forbids its graduates (M.C.D.) from advertising. Outnumbered by their less well-qualified colleagues it might have been expected that fully trained osteopaths would have aimed for a degree of unity in order to try to persuade government to legislate on the unhappy state of the profession. Instead, for many years, open hostility has existed between the three organizations, who would miss no opportunity to denigrate each other. Force of circumstances has led to a degree of co-operation being discussed, with regard, for example, to joint representation in the face of various legislative developments. One of these involves strict controls over the use of x-ray equipment, in an effort to minimize people's exposure to radiation. Desirable as this is, it has been necessary for osteopaths to attempt to ensure that their interests were taken into account in the formulation of the proposed laws. Obviously the expenses of legal advice and of a parliamentary agent are better shared, rather than duplicated by all the interested parties.

The prospect of this sort of co-operation has led to wider discussion between the three major osteopathic organizations and it is through such talks that future joint approaches to government might come. The flood of new, partly trained or untrained, practitioners has also concentrated the minds of those practitioners and their representatives who have had full time training. A united front is the only way that government agencies will be persuaded to act to sort out the current disorganized state of affairs. There have been two main attempts towards this end. The first in 1935 was initiated in the House of Lords, who appointed a select committee to look into the whole question of osteopathic recognition. At that time it was decided that the educational establishments of the day, and the profession as a whole, were too disorganized to warrent registration.

There was sympathy for the cause, but the profession was virtually told to put its house in order. To a large extent it has, insofar as it can. If the three full-time colleges and their associated organizations were to come together and seek registration it would probably succeed. However, the problem would still be, what was to be done with the 2,500 practitioners who do no fall into the category of having had a four year full-time training? This, and the rivalry between the three organizations, was the main reason for the failure of the second attempt at legislation. In 1976 Mrs Joyce Butler M.P. presented a bill to parliament under the Ten-minute rule. In her speech to the House she stated (from Hansard report, 7 April 1976):

> There is a growing interest among the general public, and even within the medical profession, in various less orthodox medical peocedures, of which osteopathy, or treatment by manipulation, is probably the best known. The interest often comes from practical experience of the success of such treatment when more usual methods have failed. Some of it is also undoubteldy a reaction against excessive drug therapy and a search for more natural methods of treatment.

She concluded by saying:

> With the growing public interest in this form of treatment it is important that it should be performed by adequately trained and experienced practitioners and that the public should be protected from those practising skills based on home study 'quickie' courses and the like, or people who may put glossy but worthless diplomas on their walls. In this country there are two training colleges for osteopathy, The British College of Naturopathy and Osteopathy and The British School of Osteopathy. Both have a full four-year course and strict entry requirements. These are recognized for student grants by the Inner London Education Authority and others. There is also the London College of Osteopathy which gives a one year course of training, to doctors. These colleges have their

own private register which intending patients can consult.

The bill which I am seeking leave to introduce proposes that there should be a statutory register of all osteopaths who have followed such a recognized course of study for a required period. The Bill will set this out in greater detail and will, I believe, be an important contribution to the status and expansion of a very important profession. It will at the same time give additional protection to the public. They can be certain that the practitioner they consult is fully qualified if his name is on this register. It is a simple and limited measure which I hope the House will approve.

Because of a failure on the part of the osteopathic organizations to agree to the proposed legislation, or to promote any common policy, the Bill was withdrawn, despite receiving an unopposed first reading. The positive results of this attempt include the fact that no opposition to the Bill was forthcoming either in or out of parliament. An editorial in the *General Practitioner* questioned whether the Bill went far enough, stating that a register, without legislation forbidding unqualified osteopaths from practising, would be insufficient. The movement towards registration will continue as the profession comes together to present a united and valid claim.

The practise of osteopathy in the U.K. is usually within a more limited range than that practised in the U.S.A. The majority of patients attending British osteopaths are suffering from obvious musculo-skeletal conditions (muscles, joints, ligaments etc.) more usually affecting the spinal column. In recent years the attitude of orthodoxy has changed dramatically. It is no longer a punishable offence for an M.D. to co-operate with an osteopath or to recommend osteopathic treatment, after decisions to this effect by the Ethical Committee of the General Medical Council. Consultant Radiographers have been given free choice as to whether or not to take, and report on, x-ray pictures for osteopath's patients. There are now osteopaths working alongside medical practitioners in the same institutions.

All this would have been impossible as recently as 1970. Public recognition of the value of osteopathic treatment has resulted in an enormous increase in the numbers of patients seeking their assistance. Many practitioners believe that osteopathic care should be freely available through the National Health Service, and if this could be organized it would greatly relieve general practitioners and hospitals. Although, since most osteopaths are already overworked, it is hard to know how they would cope. The saving in lost time to industry would be enormous; already many factories and businesses refer injured workers to osteopaths, and gladly pay their fees in the knowledge that the worker will be fit weeks earlier than otherwise. Many people cannot afford to pay for treatment, but if they live in London they can attend one of a number of clinics, such as those attached to the major colleges, where treatment is available at low cost.

Osteopathic care is more than the correction of joint problems, it is also a system of preventive medicine. By normalizing spinal and joint dysfunction before it has produced obvious symptoms, a great deal of potential trouble can be avoided. Thus, many people visit osteopaths for regular maintenance treatment and this includes assessment of young children during their vital formative years.

4. The Principles of Osteopathy

The practice of medicine and of osteopathy is an art, or skill in the application of definite rules and procedures. Such rules may, or may not, be based upon the accurate and logical interpretation of facts. If an art is based upon the logical interpretation of facts, which are understood and demonstratable, then the application of the word 'science' to the procedures is appropriate. Osteopathy is clearly an art. The clinical and practical value of osteopathic procedures is well established, but thus far there is insufficient research evidence or controlled clinical trials to produce incontravertible proof as to the validity of the theories which underlie it. This in no way invalidates the osteopathic approach.

Even if osteopathic principles cannot be scientifically proved, they do at least broaden the physician's view, and help him to look at the whole picture of the patient and his environment, which is where the skill of the physician needs to be applied, rather than simply attacking symptoms. Much research has been done, which confirms and validates osteopathic principles, and this will be discussed in the chapter on research. The aim of his chapter is to set out the basic beliefs which underlie the practice of osteopathy.

The Basic Premises

The basic premises include:

1. That the human body is an integrated unit in which structure and function are reciprocally and mutually interdependent.
2. That through complex mechanisms and systems the human body is self regulating and self healing in the face of challenges and diseases (this is known as homeostasis).

3. That optimum function of the body systems is dependent upon the unimpeded flow of blood and nerve impulses.

4. That the musculo-skeletal system comprises a major system of the body, and that its importance goes far beyond that of providing a supportive framework.

5. That there are components of disease within the structure of the musculo-skeletal system which are not only the manifestations of disease processes, but which are frequently important contributing, or maintaining, factors in disease processes. These may be local to, or distant from, such disease processes and are usually amenable to appropriate treatment

The recognition of the importance, in the overall economy of the body, of the musculo-skeletal system, its proneness to dysfunction, and the repercussions of such changes, and finally the recognition of the ability of therapy to normalize such dysfunction by one or more of a variety of manipulative procedures, represents the essence of osteopathy's individuality.

The body is functional. Structure is the manifestation of function, for structure that does not allow function is pointless. If structure alters, so will function. In a self-regulating mechanism, such as the human body, adaptation and compensation to such structural changes takes place, but always at the expense of optimum, or perfect, function. Such alterations in function may remain within acceptable limits, and not produce noticeable symptoms, but as will be seen, if these changes occur in vital spinal areas, widespread effects may take place, distant from the area of dysfunction. Structure and function should not be thought of as separate entities, one is inconceivable without the other. The musculo-skeletal system comprises roughly 60 per cent of the structure of the human body, and it expends most of the energy of the body. It has been called the 'primary machinery of life' by Professor Irvin Korr[1], who points out that our personality and our individuality are demonstrated through the musculo-skeletal system. The organs of the body can be seen as secondary, supportive, machinery, which provides energy to meet the demands of the musculo-skeletal system. It is more than just a framework which supports and contains the viscera of the body, but is the main dynamic component of the living body.

All healing systems recognize that there resides within the

body an inherent capacity for adapting to and recovering from the stress and demands placed upon it. There are many mechanisms operating towards this end. The word homeostasis is often used to describe the complex interplay of systems and processes involved in health maintenance. The hormonal, circulatory, lymphatic, nervous and musculo-skeletal systems, all interact in the maintenance and recovery of health.

Professor Korr stands out as the leading scientific researcher

Distribution of Segmental Nerves
e.g., If the roots of 1st sacral nerve are compressed pain is felt on outside of foot (the areas indicated are supplied by the nerves from the spinal level indicated by letter and number).

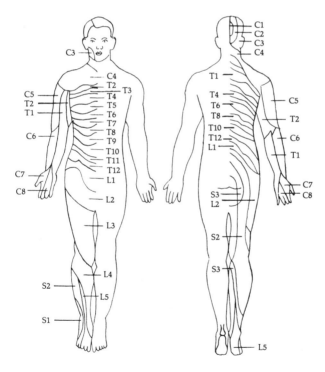

' = Cervical
  = Thoracic
  = Lumbar
  = Sacral

into the osteopathic concept. He coined the phrase 'Somatic component of disease' as far back as 1948, to conceptualize the physical entity which had previously been called the osteopathic lesion. The manner in which the musculo-skeletal system can become involved in disease processes is varied. As we shall discover, the major area through which the musculo-skeletal system influences the body, in health and disease, is through the nervous system. The body of the patient responds, through the nervous system to stimuli from its countless internal sources, as well as from external sources. The responses are mediated through the nervous system. From the neurological viewpoint, osteopathic manipulative therapy is attempting to restore function to areas of the musculo-skeletal system that are responding to increased, or abnormal, stimulation and which are modifying nerve impulses from and to the various body structures and organs. There is no part of the body that is not inter-related with every other part, via the nervous system.

A little known recent development in neurological research has shown that nerves not only carry messages but actually have a trophic function. This means that substances are transported along nerve fibres, in both directions, at varying speeds. Most of these substances are proteins and some are fats. Many degenerative diseases would appear to result from abnormalities in the transportation of these apparently vital substances along nerve pathways. We have for too long thought of the nervous system as simply a network along which impulses and messages are conducted. The implications of the nerve tissues acting as a transportation medium for essential cell substances are far-reaching.

Correct Breathing
In a more direct manner dysfunction of the musculo-skeletal system can interfere with respiratory and circulatory function. Few people realize the importance of correct breathing. Not only is this function responsible for providing the body with oxygen but it is also an important means of eliminating waste products. The effect of respiration on the circulation of blood and lymph (through the glands) is profound. As the lungs expand and contract, the diaphram rises and falls, thus altering the relative pressure between the thoracic and pelvic areas. This pump-like action is essential if venous blood is to return efficiently to the heart for re-oxygenation. The heart pumps

blood to the legs, but in order to return, the muscles of the lower extremeties need to be in use to produce the so-called 'muscle-pump' action, whereby as muscles contract they effectively squeeze the blood along the veins (which have no-return valves), and thus enable it to reach the pelvis where the diaphragmatic pump operates. If there is dysfunction in the spine which affects normal breathing, then the efficiency of blood and lymph circulation will be impaired. It is possible to appreciate, therefore, how such conditions as varicose veins and haemorrhoids can be improved by correction of body mechanics.

Unless structure is normal it cannot function normally and the consequences can be far-reaching. Goldthwait[2] states in a criticism of the medical profession, of which he was a respected member:

> Not only is little attention paid to differences in structure, but practically no consideration is given to what happens to the function of various organs, when the easily demonstrable malposition of them is considered. Is it not possible that much of what concerns chronic medicine has to do with the imperfect functioning of sagged or misplaced organs? Is it not possible that such sagging results in imperfect secretions, which at first are purely functional but if long continued may produce actual pathology? It would seem to be a matter of common sense to expect health with the body so poised or balanced that all the organs are in their proper position and the muscles in proper balance!

Korr[3] describes the manner in which the musculo-skeletal system most frequently becomes involved in disharmony:

> Man's musculo-skeletal system is an incomplete and imperfect — certainly an unstable — adaptation of a basic quadruped system to biped stance and locomotion. The components of a perfect cantilever bridge have been somewhat rearranged and modified by evolutionary process to form a less adequate skyscraper. There is no doubt that gravity is far more demanding of man's resources than of other mammalian species. As a result, local postural stresses, asymmetries, myofascial (*soft tissue*) tensions and irritations, and articular and peri-articular (*joint*) disturbances have a particularly high incidence in man. Their probability, always high, increases with time. In man, therefore, gravity has become an environmental factor of great importance.

Korr recognizes that dysfunction may result from injury, but he believes that the main cause is the result of the body's adaptation to erect posture. Individual habits, inherited factors, attitudes, occupations, the development of inborn asymetries and defects will all add to the picture, as will such factors as obesity and pregnancy. He also points out that such symptoms and signs as pain, tenderness and muscular rigidity in spinal areas, may often result from other tissues or organs which are themselves diseased or under stress, affecting spinal tissue via the nervous sytem. He states: 'Through the reciprocity of influences between visceral and somatic tissues (organs and body) via the central nervous system, visceral (organ) pathology produces disturbances in musculo-skeletal structures. This is recognized in the concept of the secondary, reflex osteopathic lesion and in the 'splinting' (muscular rigidity) associated with painful visceral (internal organ) syndromes.'

The Spinal Cord

The spinal cord is the source of most of the nerve supply to the body. Every organ and tissue receives some nerve supply which originates from the spinal cord. The cord is also the point of entry or reception of most of the information from the organs and tissues of the body. Impulses carrying information to the higher centres and the brain pass into and through the cord and are often 'screened' and organized and transmitted in, and by, tissues in the spinal cord. Everything that is happening to the body is constantly monitored and controlled via this vital pathway. Many automatic functions as well as conscious orders are either conveyed by or recoded and despatched by the cord. Insofar as the musculo-skeletal system is concerned, Korr explains it thus: [4]

> The spinal cord is the keyboard on which the brain plays when it calls for activity. But each 'key' in the console sounds not an individual 'tone' such as the contraction of a particular group of muscle fibres, but a whole 'melody' of activity, even a 'symphony' of motion. In other words, built into the cord is a large repetoire of patterns of activity, each involving the complex, harmonious, delicately balanced orchestration of the contractions and relaxation of many muscles. The brain thinks in terms of whole motions, not individual muscles. It calls, selectively, for the pre-programmed patterns in the cord and brain stem, modifying them in countless ways and combining them in an infinite variety of still more complex patterns. Each activity is subject to further modulation refinement, and adjustment by the feedback continually streaming in from the participating muscles, tendons and joints.

Since the cord is housed in a structure, the spinal column, which is patently commonly in a state of dysfunction, it is not surprising to find the perfect harmony, as described by Korr, turning into discord and disorganization. The repercussions of joint dysfunction in the spine may be local or distant. Apart from local discomfort or pain, alterations may occur in the function of nerves and their impulses and trophic functions. Whether the impulses reaching the cord are from body tissue such as muscles, ligaments, joints, etc. (somatic impulses) or from organs such as the liver, spleen etc. (visceral impulses), or whether they arise from the brain or from within the nervous system itself, such changes may be manifested in the tissues of the spinal column. The nerve cells in an area of dysfunction may become over-excited and this allow for over-reaction to stimuli. Impulses which would normally produce a small response may call forth a major one, in terms of local activity or of rapid transmission onwards of such messages. It is as though the spinal 'keyboard', because of dysfunction, was responding with a far louder note than the soft striking of a particular key warranted. Consequently disharmony results. The over-excitability of specific areas, as a result of somatic dysfunction, is known as facilitation. Professor Michael Patterson explains it thus:[5]:

> One of the most important concepts of osteopathic philosophy and practice is that of the facilitated segment. Described in research writings of the profession over the past thirty years, the concept of the facilitated segment states that because of abnormal afferent or sensory inputs to a particular area of the spinal cord, that area is kept in a state of constant increased excitation. This facilitation allows normally ineffectual, or subliminal stimuli, to become effective in producing efferent output from the facilitated segment, causing both skeletal and visceral organs inervated by the affected segment to be maintained in a state of over-activity. It is probable that the 'osteopathic lesion' or somatic dysfunction with which a facilitated segment is associated, is the direct result of the abnormal segmental activity, as well as being partly responsible for the facilitation. Although the effects of the facilitated segment on various skeletal and visceral functions are well documented, little is understood about the genesis and maintenance of spinal facilitation. Even the question of why some traumas cause facilitation and others do not, remains unanswered.

Professor Irvin Korr is the researcher whose work has led to he describing of the phenomenon of the facilitated segment and its implications. In 1955 he wrote: [6]

> Facilitation of the sensory pathways in the disturbed lesioned segments means that there is easier access to the nervous system — including the higher centres — through these segments. The lesioned segment is one through which environmental changes — especially noxious or painful stimuli — have exaggerated impact on man.
>
> Facilitation of motor pathways leads to sustained muscular tensions, exaggerated responses, postural asymmetries, and limited and painful motion. Since the muscles have rich sensory as well as motor innervation, under these conditions, they and related tendons, ligaments, joint capsules etc. may become the sources of relatively intense and unbalanced streams of impulses.
>
> The physiopathological effects of facilitation on local sympathetic pathways depend on the structures which are innerverted by those pathways; that is which viscera? which blood vessels? which glands?

The implications of an area, or areas, of the spine which is causing the various aspects of the nervous system to behave in an exaggerated manner is profound. Here is a major, perhaps the major, co-ordinating and organizing mechanism of the body, with responsibility for the defence and maintenance of life, behaving in an aberrant manner. Normally that part of the nervous system known as the sympathetic nervous system plays a vital role in organizing the adaptive and protective functions of the body. When there is sustained over-reaction on its part, damage to the organs involved, and disturbance of the entire body economy become likely. Whether or not disease results will also depend upon the total resources of the individual. Such factors as inherited tendencies, psychological balance, nutritional balance etc., all decide to some extent what physiological reserves the individual has. The facilitated segment and the havoc it causes may well be the decisive factor limiting the ability of the body to maintain itself in a disease-free state.

The work of men such as Professor Korr explains in scientific terms what the original precepts of osteopathy mean in practice. How structure and function inter-relate, how the musculo-skeletal system is capable of influencing the well-being of the body as a whole; and the implications of manipulative therapy in restoring normality. Manipulation is the means wherby areas of dysfunction are diagnosed, appraised and treated. Even when such treatment is aimed at relieving symptoms such as a backache or stiff neck, the result will be to normalize the physiological functions by reducing spinal dysfunction. Osteopathic manipulation is, therefore, best seen as a system rather than as a modality. It cannot be understood or assessed adequately outside of the context of the concepts of health and disease, from which it stems, as outlined in this chapter.

---

[1] The Sympathetic Nervous System as Mediator Between Somatic and Supportive Structures. Lecture to Postgraduate Institute of Osteopathic Medicine 1970 (New York)

[2] *Essentials of Body Mechanics,* Goldthwait, Brown, Swain and Kuhns. (J. B. Lippencott and Co.)

[3] *The Collected Papers of Irvin M. Korr.* Published by The Academy of Applied Osteopathy 1979 (first published in the Journal of the American Osteopathic Association Vol. 54 (1955)

[4] Spinal Cord as Organizer of Disease Process. 1976 Year Book of the Academy of Applied Osteopathy.

[5] [6] A model Mechanism for Spinal Segmental Facilitation by Professor Michael Patterson, 1976 Year Book of the Academy of Applied Osteopathy.

5. Diagnosis

Diagnosis of somatic dysfunction (impaired or altered function of related components of the body framework) is a relatively simple procedure when the degree of deviation from normal is marked. When, however, there is only a slight deviation, then the diagnostic exercise is more difficult. There are a variety of diagnostic methods used in assessing somatic dysfunction, and diagnostic indications fall into the following three catagories:

1. Changes in symmetry.
2. Restrictions in mobility.
3. Tissue texture changes.

The tests used to assess these changes usually fall into five classes.

1. General impression. This is a screening, either visual or by palpation (feeling by hand of the whole body or parts of it) for general asymmetries and any obvious abnormalities in structure or function. Other disciplines (physical medicine, orthopaedics etc.) use similar tests. Osteopaths tend to use their palpatory skills to focus on possible problem areas before further consideration.

2. Motion testing. A variety of tests to elicit motion, or lack of it, in regions of joint activity (e.g. low back) are utilized. These methods are not confined to osteopaths but are used in general medicine as well. Such factors as ease of movement, range of movement, continuity of movement, degreee of discomfort or pain brought about by movement, are all assessed using active (the patient moves himself), passive (the practitioner moves the patient), or resisted movements, whilst the area is palpated and 'visualized'. Restrictions in motion are noted precisely. These might include flexion, extension

sidebending or rotation limitations, for example.

3. Positional changes. The practitioner palpates for specific bony landmarks and visually judges these for asymmetry or malposition. Pairs of landmarks (shoulder blades, pelvic bones etc.) are compared and their relative positions noted. Such tests may be combined with motion tests so that position and motion can be compared simultaneously.

4. Soft tissue changes. These are assessed by inspection and palpation. Osteopathic practitioners have developed these methods to a fine art. Tissues such as muscles., ligaments and tendons are assessed for changes in temperature and consistency. The practitioner will quite likely run his hands lightly over the area being checked, seeking changes in the skin and the tissue below it. Having localized any changes in this way he will assess the deeper tissue structure by using greater pressure. He will be looking for a number of specific changes, including:

(a) *Skin changes.* Over an area of acute dysfunction the skin will feel tense and will be difficult to move, or glide, over the underlying structures.

(b) *Induration (hardening).* A slight increase in diagnostic pressure will ascertain whether or not the superficial musculature has a hardened feeling. When chronic dysfunction exists the skin and superficial musculature will demonstrate a tension and immobility, indicating fibrotic changes within and below these structures.

(c) *Temperature changes.* In acute dysfunction a localized increase in temperature may be evident. In chronic lesion conditions there may, because of relative arterial narrowing, be a reduced temperature of the skin. This usually indicates the formation of fibrous tissue in the underlying structures.

(d) *Tenderness.* Tenderness can be misleading as it may indicate local or reflex problems in acute or chronic dysfunction. The practitioner will note its presence, but not necessarily consider it as important. In acute joint dysfunction the superficial musculature and skin usually palpate as tender.

(e) *Oedema (excessive fluid).* An impression of fullness and congestion is apparent in the overlying tissues in acute dysfunction. In chronic dysfunction this has usually been replaced by fibrotic changes.

These diagnostic methods are used almost exclusively by osteopathic practitioners.

5. Local motion testing. As distinct from the testing of a region, this method attempts to assess the local response to a motion demand. The motion might be introduced by the practitioner, or the joint or area might be palpated whilst motion is introduced by the patient. Continuity of motion, tension, resistance and local tissue response are all judged. This class of tests helps to specifically identify areas of resistance to motion, and this leads to the normalizing manipulative procedures used in treatment. This is a purely osteopathic diagnostic procedure.

What Are These Tests Locating?

In the main the problems that affect general health lie in the spinal and cranial regions, as do most of the areas of dysfunction dealt with by those osteopaths whose work is confined to the aches and pains of the musculo-skeletal system. Spinal lesions display limitations of mobility, spasms of the related musculature with ligament involvement, swelling and congestion, sensitivity to pressure, and usually some degree of asymmetry. If such a state is prolonged, then chronic inflammation, fibrotic changes, contractures and arthritic changes (calcium deposits), will show themselves. Whether acute or chronic, and regardless of which of the above mentioned changes have taken place, nerve impulses will be transmitted to the central nervous system from such a lesion. These will influence other segments of the spine and affect the organs or tissues supplied from the level of the lesion. There may also, of course, be local discomfort, pain and disability.

Spinal dysfunction may also result in reflex activity from an organ to the spinal segment that supplies it. As Paul Isaacson, D.O., says:

> From a purely anatomic viewpoint, it would seem clear that a stress or strain applied to any one spinal articulation, regardless of cause, would involve several others to some degree. It would manifest itself by varying degrees of disturbance to the body mechanics, affecting posture, muscular tone, circulation, reactions to the nervous system and visceral function. At first these disturbances would be physiological, or functional, and reversible, but if allowed to persist might in time produce organic or irreversible changes in the tissues and viscera. Conversely, a primary lesion in a viscus

(organ) may predispose the musculature and ligaments, innervated by the respective segments, to lesioning.[1]

Fundamental to the successful application of any osteopathic diagnostic methods, is a highly developed tactile sense coupled with a sound knowledge of human anatomy, physiology and pathology. The ability to diagnose changes in tissue texture, symmetry and the quality and range of joint movement, presupposes a knowledge of what is normal and healthy. The experienced osteopath is able to detect changes in texture, temperature, contour and relative moisture on the surface of the skin. By palpating he can assess deeper tissue changes such as increased tension and fluid content. He can readily tell the difference betwen the state and quality of superficial and deeper muscles. By feeling and looking he can assess imbalance in structure and asymmetry and can then detect gross and subtle changes in joint mobility. This is sometimes the earliest sign of joint dysfunction.

The development of the skills required for such work involves persistent effort and practice. The osteopath must be able to receive, through the hands, the messages that are present in the tissue. These must be correctly assessed and interpreted before therapy can be meaningful or successful. Correct diagnosis is essential to successful treatment.

Dr Viola Fryman has written as follows regarding what may be discovered via palpation.[2]

1. A very light touch, even passing the hand a quarter inch above the skin, provides information on the surface temperature. An acute lesion area will be unusually warm, an area of long standing, chronic lesion may be unusually cold as compared to the skin in other areas.
2. Light touch will also reveal the cutaneous humidity, the sudorific (perspiration) or sebaceous (oily secretion) activity of the skin.
3. The tone, the elasticity, the turgor of the skin may be noted by light pressure.
4. A slightly firmer approach brings the examiner into communication with the superficial muscles to determine their tone, their fullness, their metabolic state.
5. Penetrating more deeply, similar study of the deeper muscle layers is possible.
6. The state of the fascial sheaths (fibrous tissue enveloping the muscles).
7. In the abdomen similar palpation will provide information about the state of the organs within.

8. On deeper penetration, firm yet gentle, contact is reached with bone.

Viola Fryman adds these general thoughts on palpation.

Palpation cannot be learned by reading or listening; it can only be learned by palpation. But in order to learn let us develop a perceptive, exploratory palpation; let us look to find what is under our hands, rather than seek what the text advises us should be there. Every patient, on every visit, is a new territory to be explored. A history at best incomplete. Frequently patients forget, or do not choose, to remember traumatic events. But the human body bears a record of significant injuries for the physician to read if he understands the language of the tissues. The scars of disease also remain to distort and obstruct, if the disease was supressed rather than cured. These scars must be recognized and understood. Profound emotional shock, grief and anger also leave their imprints within. The sensitive, perceptive hands can find and change these effects with lasting benefit to the patient. This is the art and science of osteopathy. [3]

Osteopathic diagnosis incorporates all that is useful and valid in standard medical diagnosis including the use of x-rays and other standard tests and procedures. These are all used as well as the unique and distinguishing measures and skills discussed above. This enables the osteopathic practitioner to read the signs that others might miss.

Knowledge of the many reflex pathways and activities in, and between, the body systems, is a further aid to accurate osteopathic diagnosis. A system which combines diagnosis and treatment is the use of what are known as neurolymphatic reflexes. These were first described by an osteopath. Dr Frank Chapman, in the 1930's. These comprise areas of 'stringy', sensitive tissue, in precise areas of the body. When present they indicate dysfunction or pathology of associated areas or organs. Treatment of these areas, by pressure techniques, is a useful method of promoting recovery, as well as being a means of ascertaining the degree of severity of the problem. There are other reflex patterns in the body such as the so called 'trigger' points (myofascial triggers) which produce pain in predictable target areas when irritated. Via knowledge of these and other reflexes, osteopaths are able to assess the patient's symptoms and can often diagnose potential problems before they have shown themselves.

[1] 'Anatomic Basis of Osteopathic Concept'. Journal American Osteopathy Association, Vol 79, No. 12, page 759.
[2] 'Palpation', Academy of Applied Osteopathy Yearbook 1963, page 17.
[3] 'Palpation', Academy of Applied Osteopathy Yearbook 1963, page 31.

6. Osteopathic Manipulation

One purpose of osteopathic manipulative therapy (OMT) is to restore physiological motion to areas in which there is restriction or dysfunction. By restoring or improving function in the musculo-skeletal system, it is anticipated that all connected parts will benefit, whether these are other parts of the musculo-skeletal system or areas influenced via nerve or circulatory pathways. OMT is not aimed at specific disease processes but rather at normalizing the musculo-skeletal structures with a view to benefiting overall function and thereby maximizing the body's homeostatic, self-regulating and healing activities.

There are a great variety of osteopathic manipulative methods. It is just as ridiculous to talk of manipulation, as though it is a specific entity, as it is to talk of medicine or surgery in the same terms. Just as the allopathic doctor, or surgeon, has a wide range of choice regarding medication or surgical procedure, so does the osteopathic practitioner have a wide range of choices regarding techniques and methods of manipulation.

Among the aims of manipulation are the restoration to normal of the supporting tissues such as muscle, ligaments, fascia etc. Then there is the normalization of movement and articulation, there is the use of reflex, mechanical, influence on the body as a whole.

Techniques can, roughly speaking, be divided into three groups:

Soft-tissue techniques. These are varied and involve any method that is directed towards tissue other than bone. Frequently soft-tissue techniques are used diagnostically, as well as therapeutically. Soft-tissue techniques may involve

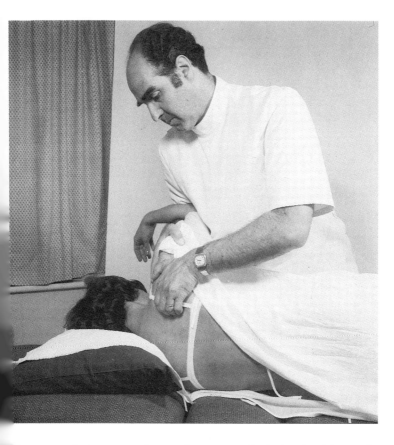

Shows a soft tissue stretching technique in which the shoulder girdle muscles are lifted and stretched. It also simultaneously allows articulation of the shoulder joint.

stretching movements across or along the lines of the muscular fibres and deep pressure techniques, as well as stretching and separation of muscle and other soft-tissue fibres, especially where muscles originate or insert into bony structures. Much soft-tissue manipulation involves working on fascia or connective tissues. These methods usually precede manipulation of the bony structures but can frequently achieve mobilization and normalization of joint structures on their own. This can result from the improvement of rigid or tense tissues, allowing a previously restricted joint to achieve a free range of motion.

A uniquely British contribution to this end was developed by the late Stanley Lief D.O., and it is in the use of this and other soft-tissue methods that attention is usually paid to the reflex areas that might influence the patient's condition. These might range from simple trigger points to more complex reflexes, involving internal function (Chapman's reflexes etc.). With soft-tissue techniques, diagnosis and treatment are often simultaneous. As the practitioner is palpating and assessing the tissues for signs of dysfunction, so is he treating and attempting to normalize what he finds.

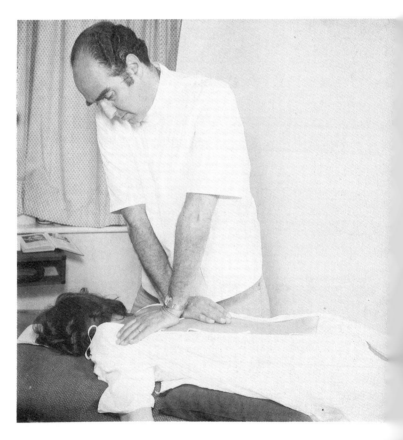

A direct action method, very similar to those employed by chiropractors. It involves high velocity and low amplitude in its execution. The supporting couch may have a sprung section to allow for a rebound effect.

Direct Techniques. In these methods the practitioner attempts to overcome limitations to normal movement by taking the joint involved towards, or through, the restrictive barrier that is preventing normal motion. This might involve thrust techniques in which, after careful positioning of the hands in relation to the joint, a high velocity, low amplitude thrusting movement forces the bony articulation to move. There would be very little movement of the hands, or of the joint in question, in such a manipulation. A matter of only a centimetre or less of actual movement might take place, but at very high speed. This

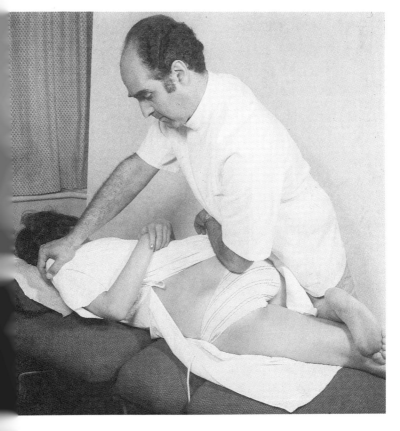

his direct action, high velocity, low amplitude manipulation involves
he precise localization of the forces required to allow correction of the
articular dysfunction. This is achieved by means of rotation and sidebending of the patient's spine, followed by the adjustment.

might be compared to trying to move a drawer that is jammed. Pushing slowly on it, however hard, will often fail to shift it, whereas a sharp tap at the appropriate angle releases it instantaneously.

A different direct method of OMT is known as articulatory technique. In this the restricted joint may be repeatedly taken through its free range, up to the point of restriction, in an attempt to gradually force a greater range of mobility, with more freedom of movement. This type of manipulation often

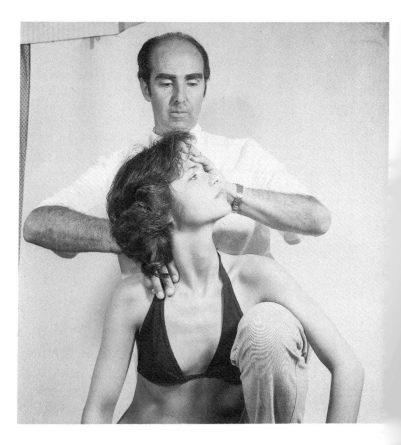

This direct action manipulation positions the patient so that by extending, side-bending and rotating the neck a locking of joint facet is obtained which localizes the forces preparatory to the high velocity low amplitude thrust being delivered to the appropriate vertebrae (in this case the second thoracic vertebrae.)

employs leverage to achieve its aims, and, as always, the longer the lever the greater the force that can be applied. A knee joint, for example, may be mobilized by the joint itself being stabilized, whilst the lower leg is grasped at the ankle and taken through a range of movements. The lower leg thus becomes a lever, and depending upon the skill with which the leverage is applied around the fulcrum (the knee joint) a great deal of controlled force can be brought to bear on the motion barriers, or on restricted tissues and surfaces. This is essentially a low velocity (slow moving), high amplitude, type of manipulation.

Muscle Energy Technique (MET) is a further method of

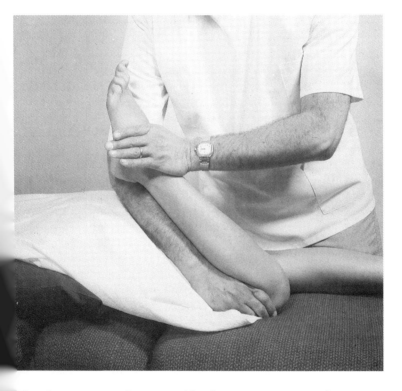

This direct action technique enables the practitioner to use leverage to force into its correct anatomical position a posterior subluxation of the head of the fibula.

applying direct action to a restricted area. With MET, however, it is the patient's own forces which produce the manipulative effort. By placing a joint in a precise position, and calling on the patient to use a muscular effort in a particular direction, against a distinctly executed counter-force from the practitioner, it is frequently possible to achieve dramatic improvements in joint mobility. The skill in such a manouevre is in creating a balance of forces which can operate precisely on the restriction. In general terms MET involves placing the joint in question at the limit of its possible motion, in the direction in which it is most restricted. This position is maintained (not exaggerated) by pressure from the practitioner and, in a controlled manner, the patient then attempts to move the joint, by sustained effort, against the practitioner's counterforce. No movement should take place during repeated short or long efforts of this type. After each such effort the joint should be reassessed, and if the range of movement has increased then the joint should be taken to this new limit before the next attempt. This method is virtually painless, and is suitable for self-use in many areas of the body (fingers or elbow, for example).

Indirect Techniques. These methods, rather than engaging and attempting (by whatever means) to overcome resistance, do the opposite. In counterstrain technique, for example, the part in question is moved by the practitioner away from the planes of restricted motion towards the planes of easier, unrestricted motion. There is a constant seeking for the position of greatest ease. At this point a mild degree of strain is introduced by the operator. This results in a reflex release of previously restricted tissues. The essence of this slowly performed technique is the introduction of the mild strain, whilst the joint is held in a position opposite to the direction in which there is a limitation of movement. It is essential that all movements are directed and controlled by the practitioner, as he eases the joint along the path of least resistance.

A further type of indirect technique is called functional technique. This also uses practitioner induced movement, whilst the area of dysfunction is constantly palpated. The joint is taken in all directions of ease (as opposed to directions of bind, which indicate irritation of tissues) gradually guiding towards the point of maximum ease. The palpating hand informs the practitioner when the affected area is least in distress. There is no further treatment at this point. The feedback from the distressed

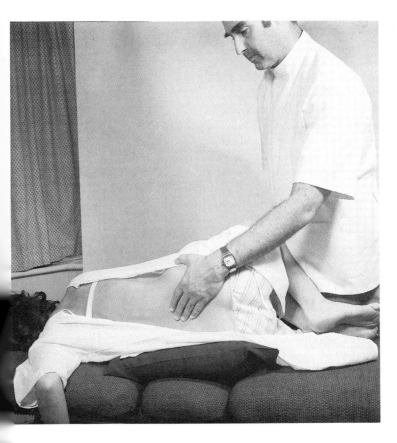

Shows the spontaneous release technique in which the affected part (in this case the low back) is carefully positioned in an exaggerated degree of the distortion already existing. This is maintained until there is a reflex release of spasm. No active manipulation is used at this usually acute stage.

joint whilst in its state of ease is enough to begin normalization.

Spontaneous release technique is a method ideally used when an area or joint is in lesion and is distorting its normal anatomical position. Often in low back problems, or neck conditions, there will be an obvious distortion. The individual might be in a stooped position or tilted to one side, or be unable to straighten a sidebent neck. This technique gently guides the affected part further into the direction of distortion. By exaggerating the lesion and holding the area in this position for several minutes, there is often a reflex release of muscular spasm and a resolution of the problem. This is a painless method.

Many techniques employ the assistance of the respiratory movements of the patient. It is a fascinating fact that as we breathe in and out, every part of the body moves. Perhaps some of the movement is very slight indeed, but it is palpable to the trained hand. For example, as we breathe in, the arms and legs rotate slightly outwards, and all the spinal joints move. The opposite (i.e. a return to the neutral position) takes place as we breathe out. Using this knowledge an osteopath will often synchronize attempts to move a joint with the phase or the respiratory cycle that will most aid the movement.

Combinations of direct and indirect techniques, sometimes preceded or followed by soft tissue methods, are often employed. Whether one method or another or a combination is needed, will be dictated by the individual case. The wide range of techniques available (and those described are by no means all) gives the osteopathic practitioner the ability to deal with musculo-skeletal problems and their ramifications.

A further area of manipulative effort is the use of cranial technique. This will be considered more closely in Chapter 11, but it is worth mentioning, in passing, that there does exist this specialized form of treatment which incorporates the cranial structures into the overall consideration of body mechanics. Cranial osteopathy attempts to normalize the bones of the head as well as influencing the circulation and fluid movements (cerebro-spinal fluid etc.) to, from and within the cranium. It attempts to balance what is known as the cranio-sacral mechanism. What this is and what its effects are will be dealt with in the appropriate chapter. The cranial concept and the techniques employed in correcting dysfunction in this area, have opened new vistas to the osteopathic profession. Birth injuries and many previously untreatable conditions have responded to cranial methods.

All osteopathic manipulation is aimed at accomplishing specific ends. Not only must the physiology of the area being treated be understood but the overall inter-relationship between it and the body as a whole needs to be considered. At the same time the manipulative techniques being employed must take into account the individual needs of the patient. When selecting the appropriate technique the practitioner visualizes the desired end result and the way in which this is most likely to be achieved. The choice will differ from patient to patient, and even in the same patient, from one visit to another.

The oldest maxim in osteopathy is 'Find it, fix it, and leave it alone'. These are golden words.

7. Research

A lot of research has been undertaken in the osteopathic field. Some relates to the way the musculo-skeletal system influences general body health and function; that is the actual changes that occur — especially in the spinal region — and the consequences of these changes. This area of research has produced great insight into the physiology and pathology of the body, whilst other research has been concerned with attempts to validate osteopathic diagnostic and therapeutic measures. This has helped to establish more clearly what is, and what is not, valid in these fields but, as with so much of research, more questions are raised as others are answered.

A major area of research was identified in the late 1930's by Dr J. Denslow, who began testing spinal dysfunction by means of pressure meters and electro-myographs (recorders of muscular contraction and relaxation). He was able to show that the areas of dysfunction required a smaller stimulus to produce muscular changes than in normal areas of the spine. In this way he demonstrated for the first time the accuracy of what had previously been the osteopath's subjective assessment through palpation that something was wrong in a particular area.

Having established that thresholds were low in areas of dysfunction, further research was needed to work out why this was so and to analyse the implications. Fortunately for osteopathy this task was undertaken by Professor Irvin M. Korr Ph.D., a biochemist and leading researcher into osteopathy who showed that when a spinal segment was in this state of over-excitability it could be stimulated, or activated, by pressure or irritation from other apparently normal segments even some distance above or below it. When the area of dysfunction was anaesthetized it could no longer be made to respond by local pressure, but would still respond to normal segments, above or below it, being pressed. At the time such troubled segments were termed 'facilitated segments'.

Professor Korr realized that pressure was, in general terms, an unnatural test of body response, and he therefore introduced other stimuli to the subject being tested, such as sudden loud noise, painful stimuli, or verbal stimuli (embarrassing questions or faked bad news). In all cases the 'facilitated segments' (the areas of lowered threshold) were the first to show a reaction, and the muscular overactivity in such regions was the last to cease when the subject relaxed. This work was reported by Korr and his associates in 1947, and he described the process as being 'like a neurological lens which focused irritation upon the lesioned segment and magnified its responses.'[1]

Investigations were then made into what was happening in such segments to the sympathetic nervous system, and the possible ramifications in the body as a whole. This involved mapping the patient's skin surface for variations in electrical resistance and temperature. This produced a visual record of the sympathetic nervous system behaviour, as reflected by sweat gland activity and blood flow, under the skin, of any given area at a particular moment in time.

This system has been superceded by infra-red photography as well as by the use of sophisticated electronic apparatus which simultaneously measures eight different spinal segments. All this has proved that there exists a correlation between the lesioned segment (area of somatic dysfunction) and the abnormal behaviour of motor and sympathetic nerves that are segmentally related to the lesioned area.

Patterns of Dysfunction

Over the years Korr began to establish consistent patterns of sympathetic nerve function disturbances and specific organ diseases, especially where pain was a major factor, such as pancreatitis, peptic ulcer, gall bladder disease, menstrual pain, colic, kidney stones etc. Often students who had volunteered for assessment were noted as having patterns of dysfunction which later would show up as a specific disease pattern.

Professor Korr admits that much work in this field remains to be done, but he states that when a condition of chronic facilitation exists in a spinal segment, 'We cannot say that this 24-hours-a-day state of alarm results in illness on a definite one-to-one basis. We can only say that these disturbed segments are relatively vulnerable, that the probability is higher. Whether or not it becomes clinically significant depends upon the person we are dealing with and all the circumstances of his life, past, present and future. Here is where other unfavourable circumstances in the patient's daily life may tip the balance; here is where an abnormal stress response will tend to find the earliest and most severe expression.'[2]

In addition to this line of research Professor Korr has done much work on the trophic function of nerves (concerning the nutrition of the tissues). Nerves not only conduct impulses but supply proteins and other substances to the tissues and organs with which they connect. These substances are essential for the maintenance and self-repair of the tissues, and they influence their total function. In considering the implications of this, Korr states that any factors that interfere with this aspect of nerve function may contribute towards disease. He says:

> Such factors could include disturbances (e.g. emotional stress) in descending impulse traffic from higher centers, impulse traffic in sensory pathways from various parts of the body, nutritional factors, drugs, toxicological agents, viral insults, changes in the chemical environment of the neurons and their axons (nerve cells) and, of course, the mechanical stresses and large forces exerted on and generated by the myofascio-skeletal tissues through which the nerves pass, and the accompanying chemical changes in these tissues. It seems likely that the efficacy of manipulative therapy may occur in part through alleviation of some of these detrimental factors.

More recently it has been shown that the flow of material along nerves is a two-way traffic. The retrograde transport is seen as a means of communication, or feedback (literally) between the nerve cells and the cells they supply. Korr states:

> Any factor that causes derangement of transport mechanisms in the axon or that chronically alters the quality or quantity of the axonally transported substances, could cause the trophic influence to become detrimental. This alteration in turn would produce aberrations of structure, function and metabolism, thereby contributing to dysfunction and disease.
>
> Almost certainly to be included among these harmful factors is the deformation of nerves and roots, such as compression, stretching, angulation and torsion, that are known to occur all too commonly in the human being, and that are likely to disturb the

intra-axonal [nerve cell process] transport mechanisms, intra-neural [nerve cell] micro-circulation [circulation in the smallest blood vessels] and the blood-nerve barrier. Neural structures are especially vulnerable in their passage over highly mobile joints, through bony canals, intervertebral foramina [apertures], fascial layers [fibrous tissue beneath the skin] and tonically contracted muscles (for example, posterior rami [branches] of spinal nerves and spinal extensor [stretching] muscles.) Many of these biochemically induced deformations are, of course, subject to manipulative amelioration and correction. [3]

As Paul Thomas D.O. states:

This appears to be a part of the long sought answer to the question of exactly how the nerves influence the structures innervated, with respect to metabolism, development, differentiation, regeneration, and trophicity in general. The treatment of an organ through its innervation is an element in present manipulative therapy. The new information regarding neural function may lead to specific improvements in technique. [4]

This knowledge, plus the segmental facilitation research of Korr and his associates, gives a scientific basis for the claims of osteopathic medicine; i.e. that dysfunction of the musculo-skeletal framework of the body can have profound effects on the health of the individual.

Research Into Diagnostic Methods

Research into the ability of osteopathic diagnostic methods to elicit accurately such dysfunction has also been carried out and evaluated. Between 1969 and 1972 over 6,000 patients admitted to Chicago Osteopathic Hospital were part of just such a clinical investigation. Visual and palpatory observations made by attending osteopathic physicians were recorded and analysed in relation to the health problems of the patients. The findings showed a clear link between the spinal area, diagnosed by the examining practitioner as being involved, and the corresponding diseased organs of the patient. The conclusion was: 'The somatic findings in over 6,000 cases of hospital patients support the osteopathic theory of viscero-somatic (internal organs and the body) relationships.' [5]

In clinical situations a variety of findings over the years have tended to validate the osteopathic concept. One such investigation related to the study of the relationship between disorders of the pelvic and thoracic organs, and spinal findings.

It was ascertained that the following three palpable findings occurred in statistically significant numbers of tests:

Restricted intervertebral motion occurring alone.

Restricted intervertebral motion occurring in combination with abnormal vertebral position.

Restricted intervertebral motion occurring in combination with abnormal paravertebral musculature.

The cases assessed were of uncomplicated disorders of the heart, aorta, bronchii and lungs (86 cases) and disorders of the female genitalia (101 cases).

Research was carried out in 1965 at Los Angeles County Osteopathic Hospital into the effects of osteopathic care of children with pneumonia.[6] Here 239 cases of various types of pneumonia in children over a three year period were analysed. The results showed that there was a favourable comparison with results of treatment in non-osteopathic institutions of a similar nature.

Around the same time research was also conducted into the possibility of a musculo-skeletal connection in cases of cardiac disorder, and the results yielded strong evidence of such a correlation.[7] Palpatory, and x-ray findings, as well as prior fluoroscopic and E.C.G. readings, showed that a majority of the 150 patients in the tests had associated asymmetrical spiral aberrations and corrective spinal treatment was consistently found to be followed by varying degrees of relief from cardiac symptoms. These changes were reflected in objective clinical and laboratory tests.

More recently, in 1981, doctors at Riverside Osteopathic Hospital in Trenton, Michegan, undertook an investigation to establish the existence of a viscero-somatic reflex that could be easily detectable and which would correlate with the presence of athero-sclerotic coronary artery disease. In all, 88 consecutive cases, each suggesting coronary disease, underwent cardiac catheterization, and within one week of this, each patient in turn was given standard osteopathic musculo-skeletal evaluation (pain, range of movement, soft tissue texture etc.) by an examiner unaware of the results of the cardiac catheter probe. The results showed a correlation between coronary athero-sclerosis and abnormalities of range of motion and soft tissue texture in the fourth and fifth thoracic and the third cervical intervertebral segments.[8]

At the same time research at the Philadelphia College of

Osteopathic Medicine demonstrated that there occurs a definite, measurable and significant drop in the intraocular pressure following osteopathic manipulative therapy.[9] This is of great significance to patients with chronic open angle glaucoma.

Such research efforts are constantly being undertaken to establish the value of osteopathic treatment, and the fundamental and far-reaching results obtained by Professor Korr and others, as well as the cumulative evidence of many groups and individuals in the clinical field, have gone a long way towards this end already.

[1] 'The Neural Basis of the Osteopathic Lesion', *The Journal of the American Osteopathic Association* 47: 191-198 (1947).

[2] 'The Trophic Function of Nerves and Their Mechanisms', *The Journal of the American Osteopathic Association* 72:163-171 (1972).

[3] 'The Spinal Cord as Organizer of Disease Processes', *The Journal of the American Osteopathic Association*, Vol. 80, No. 7, page 458.

[4] *Osteopathic Medicine*, Hoag, Cole and Bradford (McGraw Hill 1969).

[5] 'A Clinical Investigation of the Osteopathic Examination', Kelso, Larson and Kappler, *The Journal of the American Osteopathic Association*, Vol. 79, No. 7, page 460.

[6] 'Pneumonia Research in Children at L.A.C. Osteopathic Hospital', Warson and Percival, *Yearbook of the Academy of Applied Osteopathy*, 1965, page 152.

[7] 'A Somatic Component in Heart Disease', Richard Koch D.O., *The Journal of the American Osteopathic Association*, May 1961.

[8] 'Palpatory Musculo-skeletal Findings in Coronary Artery Disease: Results of a Double Blind Study', Cox, Rogers, Gorbis, Dick and Rogers, *The Journal of the American Osteopathic Association*, July 1981.

[9] 'Evaluation of Intraocular Tension Following Osteopathic Manipulative Therapy', Paul Misischia D.O., *The Journal of the American Osteopathic Association*, July 1981.

8. Osteopathy in Practice

Most patients consulting osteopathic practitioners will do so in the hope of obtaining relief from musculo-skeletal aches and pains. In the main, the low back and neck are the areas most likely to be involved, but all the joints and muscles of the body are possible sources of problems which may be helped by osteopathic care. A growing number of patients, however, do consult osteopaths about a wider range of health problems, and these might include such conditions as migraine headaches, tinnitus (noises in the head), dizziness, bronchial problems, asthma, functional cardiac problems, digestive problems and menstrual irregularities. The treating of these and other conditions by osteopathic methods can be surprisingly successful.

What Happens On Visiting an Osteopath

A typical visit to an osteopath can last from fifteen to forty-five minutes, depending upon the condition, and at the first visit the osteopath will take a case history and conduct a detailed examination and assessment of the spinal and other joints. Should the condition warrant it, x-ray pictures might be taken. In many cases the heart and chest will be examined, blood pressure taken and possibly other clinical tests performed or arranged (urine tests, blood tests, eye or ear assessments etc.). In these ways the osteopath arrives at a diagnosis as to the causes of the patient's problems, or at least as to the possible musculo-skeletal involvement in whatever problem the patient is troubled with.

Treatment normally consists of preliminary soft-tissue manipulation. This might be local to the area of pain, or distant from it if the osteopath is attempting to influence the condition reflexly. Having stretched, relaxed and generally prepared the soft tissues, the osteopath will manipulate the appropriate joint or joints. As shown in Chapter 6, a variety of methods may be used at this stage. The age, condition, degree of pain and spasm etc. will all decide which is the most desirable approach.

Some forms of manipulation produce an audible snapping or

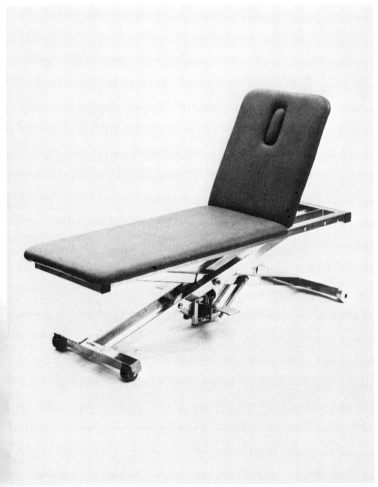

Photo: Courtesy Rehabilitation Products Limited

An osteopathic treatment couch.

popping sound. This is thought to result from the creation of a momentary vacuum between the joint surfaces as they are manipulated. Such sounds do not necessarily indicate that the manipulation has been successful, nor does the absence of such sounds mean that the treatment has failed to achieve mobility.

After treatment there is often immediate relief from pain and improved mobility. However, there may be a degree of transient discomfort, and in some cases a slight increase in pain may be felt for a day or so, especially in acute conditions. More usually there is a feeling of well-being. Some patients experience a marked degree of relaxation and a desire to sleep, and others feel a sense of exhilaration and energy.

Practitioners will explain the objectives of the treatment, and may well suggest a programme of home treatment to augment and support the osteopathic therapy. This could include exercise, dietary changes and relaxation. If the condition is a simple mechanical strain, then it would normally be correctable fairly quickly, and require no further attention. If, on the other hand, the condition is of a more chronic nature, then periodic maintenance treatment may be necessary to prevent a recurrence.

The frequency of osteopathic treatment can vary from very often, say every other day, to occasional, say every month or so. In chronic conditions the regular 'maintenance' treatment is likely to be at intervals of anything from once weekly to once in three or four months. There is a tendency for patients to be advised to have regular check-ups, two or three times a year, on the same basis as in dentistry. Since many minute musculo-skeletal changes often precede obvious problems by many months, this preventive approach can be of value. In the same way an increasing number of infants and growing children are taken for osteopathic assessments each year to ensure that problems are corrected before they become established.

Many patients speak of their problems in terms of 'bones being out of place'. They therefore expect these to be replaced or 'put back' by manipulation. Such ideas are largely inaccurate and over-simplistic. Whilst slight changes in position may take place, the essence of osteopathic manipulation is the restoration of mobility between joint surfaces. Correction of positional lesions tends to be achieved by normalizing the soft tissues that are supporting, binding and holding the bones in their particular positions. Some individuals have hypermobile joints due to congenital or acquired ligamentous weakness. Such joints can become unstable and, far from requiring manipulation, may need stabilizing by improvement of the tone of the soft tissues. This is sometimes achieved by injecting a sclerosing agent which 'tightens' the supporting tissues.

The 'Slipped Disc'

The commonest diagnosis with which patients arrive at an osteopaths door (in the UK) is that of a slipped disc. Very few doctors have studied the mechanics of the spine with the degree of detail required of the qualified osteopath. The most common diagnosis given in cases of acute low back pain is that of a 'slipped disc'. The symptoms vary, but usually involve stabbing pain on movements, and often one-sided spasm of the lumbar muscles; there is great difficulty in standing erect, and there may be pain down one or both legs. These symptoms are usually present in a true case of prolapsed intervertebral disc, but may be present in any other conditions. How is one to know?

A detailed history of the onset will often enable a correct diagnosis to be made and with details of the past medical history and a careful physical examination, it is possible to confirm or rule out the diagnosis of a slipped disc, with a great degree of certainty.

For the unfortunate individual suffering from a strained sacro-iliac joint, who is told by his doctor that he is suffering from a 'slipped disc', life becomes very irksome. He may be put to bed for anything up to six weeks, and then put into a corset. He may find himself in a plaster cast or in some cases an operation is suggested. If the patient is really suffering from a prolapsed disc ,the period in bed or wearing the corset would rest the area and enable a degree of repair to take place, but if the trouble is a strain of the sacro-iliac joint these treatments would be worse than useless.

The disc that it supposed to slip is a tough cartilaginous ring that is firmly attached to the vertebrae above and below it. This contains an inner pulpy mass, the *nucleus pulposis.* When through strain or an injury a tear appears in the cartilage, the inner material can protrude. This will cause spasm in the surrounding musculature and if there is pressure on nerves in the area then there will be acute pain. The disc does not, indeed cannot 'slip'. There can be a rupture, or a herniation, and thus the misnamed 'slipped disc.'

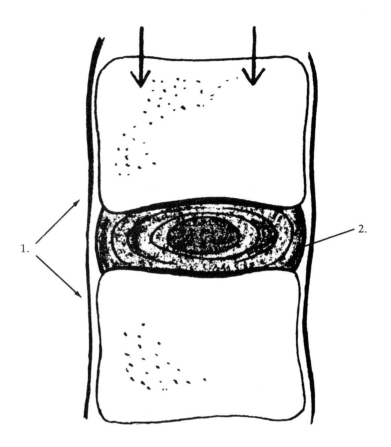

Cross Section of: 1. Vertebral Bodies
Showing: 2. Disc in healthy state.

The effect of long-term unnatural wear on the disc is to reduce
the elasticity of the disc as a whole and to produce a narrowing,
degenerative change. Thus the ability of the disc to act as a
shock-absorber becomes reduced. This results in stiffness and
loss of mobility and possibly pain. It is therefore apparent that
anything that can be done to prevent this all too common
degeneration is highly desirable.

Once a disc has herniated there is no way of 'putting it back.'
Anyone who claims to replace a 'slipped disc' is, without doubt,
not being accurate. It is possible, with manipulation, to ease the
pressure on the disc, then with gentle exercise and care the slow

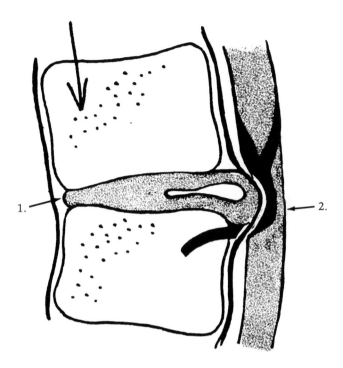

Cross Section Showing: 1. Prolapsed Disc with: 2. Pressure on Nerve Root. Such a condition would produce sciatic pain if this occurred in the Lumbar Spine.

repair can take place. In rare cases surgery may be needed to remove the extruded pulp, but I would suggest that surgery should never be resorted to before an osteopath has been consulted.

Whether short-term painful joint problems, or long-term general health conditions are the reason for consulting an osteopath, the way the individual uses his body will to a large extent determine whether or not recurrence of the problem takes place. For this reason it is vital that after correction of areas of dysfunction, the patient be instructed in the correct use of the body and in appropriate exercises. Many osteopaths also advise their patients on correct nutrition and in this way provide a comprehensive health care service.

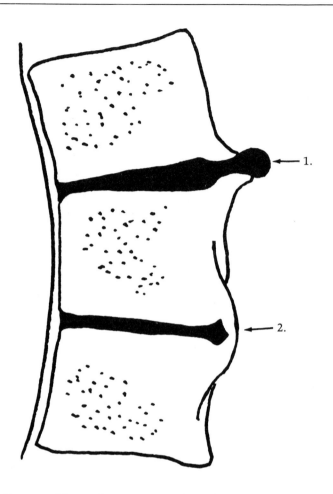

Cross Section of Spine showing: 1. Prolapsed Disc; 2. Bone Degeneration.

Other Complaints Which Osteopathy May Help
Without attempting to cover all the possible disease states that osteopathic manipulative therapy might be able to help. I list below a selection of examples with the idea of giving some idea of osteopathy's possibilities.

Allergic Conditions
The treatment of causes rather than symptoms is of first

importance, and a lot of attention will need to be given to both the nutritional and stress related aspects of the problem. There are, though, quite often cases where osteopathic manipulation can help. In asthma, for example, areas of dysfunction may be found around the second thoracic vertebra, and there are always restrictions in the normal range of movement of the ribs. Such structural problems may be improved or corrected by osteopathic treatment, but if nothing is done about the underlying hormonal, nutritional and stress factors there is a strong likelihood that the allergy will reappear.

In most cases of allergy there is a degree of adrenal gland dysfunction (inadequate adrenaline production in response to repeated stress arousal, for example) or liver dysfunction (inadequate production of anti-hystamine in response to allergic hystamine production). Both these organs can be to some extent adversely affected over a period of time by mechanical disorders in the spine, and spinal correction through osteopathic manipulation can sometimes bring about an improvement of function.

Arthritis
The localized degenerative changes to joints which are collectively labelled osteo-arthritis or osteo-arthrosis is afflict the majority of people over 35 who live in industrialized countries, and the term 'wear and tear' adequately describes the joint damage which results from the misuse of the postural and weight-bearing joints such as the spine, hips, knees etc.

In the early stages of such wear and tear, when disability is first becoming apparent in the form of stiffness, discomfort and slight limitation of movement, it is possible through osteopathic manipulative treatment to halt, and perhaps even reverse, the initial damage to the soft tissues which precedes the actual joint surface damage.

Even in cases of existing osteo-arthritic conditions, improvement may be brought about through osteopathic treatment in terms of improved mobility, the lessening of pain, and possibly the slowing down of the degenerative process. This is especially likely in spinal regions such as the neck and upper thortic spine and the lower back and pelvic joints which are those most abused by bad postural habits. Osteopathic treatment cannot undo the damage already done, however, but it can often minimize the effects by increasing the degree of mobility in all but extremely advanced cases.

Bronchitis

Chronic or acute obstruction of the breathing passages may yield to osteopathic manipulative therapy, although the causative factors must also be dealt with, and it is not suggested that structural factors play a major part in the background to bronchitic conditions. Osteopathic treatment in the spinal, chest and diaphragm areas can improve respiratory function and seems to speed the elimination of obstructing mucus. Apart from the mobilizing of the structure of the chest, such as ribs and their articulations with the spine and sternum, there are specific osteopathic methods such as the 'thoracic pump' and the 'diaphragmatic doming' techniques which may help.

Constipation

When the problem results from an over-contracted or spastic bowel, osteopathic treatment may assist in normalizing the condition, in conjunction with a restructured diet to include a high degree of fibre.

Digestive Complaints

Osteopaths find that there is frequently a spinal element involved in digestive dysfunction, whether the condition involves over- or under-supply of acid, or over- or under-supply of enzymes, or increased or decreased blood supply, to particular regions of the digestive organs. Osteopathic treatment is non-specific in such conditions, and usually areas of spinal dysfunction will be found in the mid and lower thoracic areas. The normalizing of these, together with dietary changes, can alleviate the problem.

Headaches

There are a great variety of causes of what are generally termed headaches, but one of the main causes of the common headache is tension in the neck and back of the skull and this is found to be particularly amenable to osteopathic treatment. Also, a definite reduction in frequency and intensity of pain was found to result from the osteopathic normalization of the cervical spine when research into migraine was conducted at the British College of Naturopathy and Osteopathy in the early 1970s.

Many headaches of less obvious origins may respond to a combination of cranial, cervical and upper thoracic normalization, but it would be wrong to assume that all headaches can always be relieved by osteopathy. In my own experience, however, I have found that some headaches of many years duration have yielded to just one treatment session.

Heart Conditions

Generally the improvement of mobility in the thoracic spine and chest region after osteopathic manipulation seems to enhance the heart's function and in turn the blood is more efficiently oxygenated.

References have been made in Chapter 7 to the results of research into the possibility of a musculo-skeletal connection in cases of cardiac disorder, and the correction of spinal dysfunction by osteopathic manipulative therapy is claimed to reduce the chances of cardiac distress.

A frequent finding is that of what has come to be called 'false angina'. In this condition all the classical symptoms of angina occur (pressure in the chest, breathlessness, pain in one or both arms etc.) but they fail to respond to drug therapy. In many such cases there is found to be an upper thoracic lesion which responds to simple manipulative techniques with a consequent disappearance of the symptoms.

Hiatus Hernia

This distressing condition involves a bulging upwards, through a gap in the diaphragm, of part of the stomach. Osteopathy's normalizing treatment of the structures to which the diaphragm attaches itself can be of great assistance, and there are also soft tissue manipulations which can be applied direct to the diaphragm, the muscles of the abdomen and the stomach itself. By thus improving the mechanics affecting the diaphragm, as well as the other factors involved in the problem, the distressing symptoms of hiatus hernia may be minimized. Other factors, such as obesity, bad posture, stress and poor nutrition, must not be overlooked, but osteopathy can in a number of cases be decisive in relieving symptoms and helping to correct the mechanical strain which allows the initial upwards displacement of the stomach.

Hypertension

If high blood pressure is the result of tension then osteopathic manipulative therapy can have a very beneficial effect on the condition. Both research and clinical experience shows that the normalization of spinal and general mechanics seems to have a stabilizing effect on the systolic and diastolic readings for a number of weeks. It is not suggested, though, that osteopathy should be used as the major method for treating hypertension, but such treatment can be a useful additional therapy.

Menstrual Problems

Dramatic improvements in menstrual function, in terms of regularity, less pain and discomfort, and shorter periods, have been achieved through the normalization of dysfunction of the lumbo-sacral area of the spine. There are many possible contributory factors in menstrual problems. Some of these are hormonal, others emotional, and others involve nutritional imbalances. However, in many cases the cause of the problem lies in mechanical and postural factors. In some cases there is a marked increase in the angulation of the lumbar spine causing a hollow, or 'sway', back and this can result in the pelvic organs being literally tilted forward and crowded into the lower pelvis. This can be helped toward a more normal position by osteopathic treatment.

Sciatica

If there is a pain radiating down the leg, then it may be the result of some degree of nerve root irritation involving the sciatic nerve. Some forms of this condition are not amenable to osteopathic care; for example, when the nerve is actually inflamed (neuritis). However, in the majority of cases of sciatica the nerve is irritated and not inflamed (neuralgia) and in many such cases removal of the cause of the irritation by osteopathic treatment relieves the pain. The cause may lie in the low back or in the pelvic or buttock regions. In acute cases it may be the result of a prolapsed disc, in which case osteopathy may be of only limited value.

Tinnitus

This intensely aggravating condition, which involves a ringing buzzing or hissing sound in the ears, can be relieved by cranial manipulation.

9. The Effects of Stress

Stress of a psychological or emotional nature can produce marked changes in the musculo-skeletal system, profoundly influencing the overall functioning of the body. All emotional changes are mirrored in the soft tissues. Attitudes such as anger or fear, as well as moods such as excitement or depression, produce muscular postures and patterns. There is also a close link between habitual posture and psychological attitudes and states.

Many postures and defensive tensions arise from anxiety and stress. If this is continued and repeated, restrictions and alterations will take place in the soft tissues. If unreleased these become self-perpetuating and the source of pain and of more stress. The ability to relax is frequently lost and the consequent drain on nervous energy is marked.

The unique understanding which osteopathy brings to the way in which the body functions helps to clarify the manner in which stresses can produce quite different effects in different people.

Have you ever focused sunlight through a magnifying glass to obtain a pinpoint of heat? If, in this metaphor, stress, in all its myriad forms, is represented by the light of the sun, then the focusing mechanism (the lens) is represented by the nervous system. Our attention must be on both aspects of this phenomenon, the stress factors, and how to avoid or minimize them, and the body systems which deal with stress, and in particular the nervous system, which to a large extent determines how the body will cope with it. No two people react to stress in the same way. Even under identical conditions, reactions and effects will vary. While it is important to know what stress is, and how the body reacts to it in general, more attention should be applied to the individual receiving the stress, the unique characteristics of whom will determine the end result.

Why does one person develop an ulcer, another diabetes and yet another high blood pressure? All these conditions might be the apparent result of similar stress patterns. It is obvious, therefore, that the stress factors do not themselves determine the response of the body. The unique make up and history of the individual is the determining factor in deciding just what aspects of the body will adapt or react in response to any stimulus or stress. Disease in the final analysis is the failure, on the part of the body, to adapt to, or cope with, the demands placed upon it by the total environment in which it lives. This includes demands of a stressful nature, whether internally generated or externally applied.

The 'Fight or Flight' Response

Stress is a word which is glibly used and which is often misused. It does not in fact have a single meaning, for it can encompass any real or potential stimulus, usually (but not always), of a noxious or unpleasant nature, to which the body or mind is subjected. This might include such varied factors as intense heat or cold, negative emotional states, inadequate nutrition, excessive noise, fear, drugs, polution, pain, etc. Much stress is exogenous, that is it comes from outside the body, but it may often be endogenous, i.e. it is self-generated (hate, envy, fear, jealousy etc). Any stress factor can be the apparent cause of the reactions on the part of the mind/body complex of the individual. Such reactions are often described in terms of the 'fight or flight' response. This describes the primitive response to danger in which immediate preparation is made by the body to defend itself (fight) or run away (flight). The generally accepted reasoning is that since such responses are often socially unacceptable (it is not done to hit out physically or to run away in most stressful situations) the various physiological responses which accompany arousal to fight or flight become, with repetition, the apparent cause of a great deal of physical and mental ill health. A large number of physical changes take place at times of stress induced arousal. These include: the brain and nervous system becomes intensely active, the pupils of the eyes dilate, there is a slowing of the digestive process (which usually stops) the saliva stops and the mouth becomes dry, muscle tense in preparation for activity and the heart pumps blood harder and faster in anticipation of the extra activity; blood pressure rises; breathing becomes faster, to the point of gasping; hormones such as adrenaline are released into the system, as is glucose (from the liver); sweating commences in response to the need to cool the body etc. All this and more is accomplished in a split second under the direction and control of the nervous system.

If the stress factors are rapidly removed then no harm is done and all the changes are reversed. Equally, if a valid response, of a fight or flight nature, is forthcoming (running away from an angry dog or punching a potential mugger) then the physiological changes will have been used appropriately, and normality will return. Such responses are, however, not appropriate to most modern stress situations (unhappy marriage, financial anxieties, fear of redundancy etc.) and if stress factors are constant, or repeated frequently, and there is no release of the build-up of tension, or adequate rest phase from the physiological changes described, then a variety of symptoms can show themselves, including dizziness; stiff aching muscles; headache; visual problems; hypertension; circulatory and heart problems; breathing difficulties, including asthma; allergies; palpitations; digestive disorders, including ulcers; swallowing difficulties; blood sugar irregularities (high or low); backache; skin disorders; bowel disorders (constipation or colitis); sexual difficulties etc.

All these can result from other causes, of course, but often appear when there is prolonged exposure to stress. Noxious stress factors often fall into categories such as difficult personal relationships; excessive pressure due to deadlines and time factors; financial anxiety; inability to communicate deeply held feelings or resentment; personality problems (self doubt etc.), inability to focus and live in present time (the future or past dominate); dramatic life style changes etc.

Stress is not always noxious, or unpleasant but, as defined by modern clinicians, includes many apparently pleasant events, and is now seen to include almost anything, good or bad, which alters the status quo. An outstanding personal achievement, for example, is seen to create as much stress as a change in responsibility at work. A holiday such as Christmas is seen as being equally stressful to the receiving of a parking ticket. Change, itself, is seen as requiring a response, or adaptive change, on the part of the individual, and this is regarded as stressful. Much stress is indeed health enhancing and life enriching, and, indeed, without a degree of arousal we would be cabbage-like in our existence.

General Adaptation Syndrome

When stress is prolonged, or repeated frequently, though, a series of changes may begin which are part of what is known as the General Adaptation Syndrome (G.A.S.). Initially the self-regulating mechanisms of the body, which maintain internal balance, or homeostasis, cope adequately with the constant episodes of arousal, with all the changes that these call for. Eventually, after months or years though, the ability of one aspect or another of the body to adapt, or cope adequately, will become impaired. Imbalance and breakdown of internal balance begins, and the exhaustion stage of the G.A.S. takes over from the adaptive stage. This is when unpleasant symptoms become noticeable. Depending upon the very personal, and unique, attributes of the individual's physiological and psychological make-up, the way this exhaustion stage manifests itself will vary.

The signs of stress become apparent, and anything from insomnia to asthma, to high blood-pressure, to exhaustion or depression or ulcers may result. If treatment at this stage is aimed at these symptoms then little good can be expected to result. The only real hope is to deal with causes and this involves both the stress factor, and the body and mind, of the individual. This is the holistic concept which permeates 'natural healing' in general and osteopathy in particular. If nothing positive is done during the exhaustion phase of the G.A.S. then final break-down and death will eventually result. If treatment is palliative (drugs etc.), then a similar end-result should be anticipated, although the symptoms might be made more bearable for a while. If, however, the 'total' picture is dealt with, there is hope of recovery to optimum health. In dealing with stress *all* aspects need attention. Primarily the life style of the individual requires an overhaul. How much rest? relaxation? meditation? Is the diet balanced and does it include an adequate amount of vital nutrients? What aspects of the stress problem can be helped by counselling? by psychotherapy? by gaining insights?

It is known that if a 'stressed' individual can be placed on an optimum diet and be encouraged to exercise regularly, to take regular and adequate rest, then many 'diseases' of stress simply go away. If, at the same time, other aspects of the individual's life style (attitudes, amount of work undertaken, personality traits etc.) can be modified, then even more improvement can be expected. It is interesting to know that it is quite possible for an aggressive, compulsively hard working, individual to change into a relaxed and carefree one, by the altering of attitudes and behaviour. The statement 'that's how I am, I'm afraid', is meaningless — we *can* change if it matters enough.

Spinal Dysfunction

What is it that determines which part of the body will break down under prolonged stress?. There are inherited tendencies of course and this must be borne in mind. There is another key 'organizer' within the body, to which the osteopathic profession, in particular, pays much attention. This is the nervous system and the role of spinal dysfunction in affecting the way in which particular patterns of ill-health are manifested. Extensive research in the U.S.A., much of this conducted by Professor Irvin Korr over the past 35 years has established the following:

1. That there exists in most people's spines, areas, or segments, which are abnormal or aberrant in one of (at least) three ways. These areas may be hypersensitive to pressure; restricted in mobility (movement) or asymmetrical (out of position). Such changes are common, even in apparently healthy people.

2. These areas are abnormal in the degree of tension or tone that is present in the local soft tissues, and the nerves in such an area respond abnormally to any stimulus. Some of the nerve cells which deal with messages of sensation, or which direct automatic function, or which direct voluntary function, will be in a state of chronic over-excitability. In other words they will react more rapidly and more strongly, and for longer, than they should, to even a mild stimulus *of any sort*.

3. This state of over-reaction is often manifested in the tissues or organs which these nerve cells supply, or control.

These abnormally reacting segments may result from injury, or postural stress, or they may result from problems in a particular organ or system (say a diseased gall bladder) which feeds back 'irritable' messages along the nerves supplying it, to the spinal centres, where local irritation may become chronic and cause changes in the tone of the soft tissue. Whether the initial cause is reflex (from the organ to the spinal area) or direct, i.e. biomechanical changes in the spine itself, the result is an over-reacting segment of the nervous system. Since the nervous system organizes the body's adaptive and protective functions, in dealing with all environmental variations and extremes (changes of temperature, increased activity etc.), as well as its reaction to emotional stress (alarm reaction etc.), such a state of over-excitability, in a particular area, has enormous local and distant consequences.

Instead of, for example an organ being controlled in a balanced harmonious way, it might be kept in a state of near constant over-(or under-) stimulation, because the nerve centres controlling its function are in this condition. As previously mentioned, such an area is known as a facilitated segment (i.e. it allows easier conduction of nerve impulses and activity). These result in unpredictable effects on the target organ. If such an area occurs in the upper spinal region it might be associated, for example, with heart dysfunction. A definite pattern of spinal lesion has been found in most cases of angina pectoris (severe constricting pain in the chest). If, in a mid-spinal area, then the effect might be on the digestive organs such as the liver or pancreas etc. Now, it must be remembered that although the spinal area is maintaining such over-, or under-, activity via the nervous system, the problem might have originated in the organ itself, for a variety of reasons (infection, toxic state etc.), and the spinal irritation and consequent facilitated state might originally have resulted from this.

If stress is part of the individual's life, then the presence in the spine of such areas, and they are the rule rather than the exception, will cause over-reaction, in a chronic manner and the end result will be that the target organ or system will become abnormal in its function. In the fullness of time this, unchecked, will result in damage and dysfunction of the affected organ and disturbance of the entire body economy.

Osteopathic methods enable practitioners to speedily identify such 'facilitated' or lesioned segments, Osteopathic manipulation of the spine and soft tissues (e.g. neuro-muscular technique) can often normalize these areas, but in chronic cases only limited improvement may be possible.

All controllable factors in, and around, any ill person should be the concern of whoever is treating them. This should take account of the whole life style and personality of the individual. After balancing the obvious factors (sleep, relaxation, exercise, diet, etc.) there still remains the normalizing of the biomechanical component of the body, the musculo-skeletal system in general and the spine in particular. Stress can be seen in this light to cause, and perpetuate, dysfunction and disease, in direct proportion to the individual's unique make-up, both mental and physical. Osteopathy presents the opportunity to intervene by helping to normalize the very structures which 'organize' the effects of stress on the body. This, together with counselling regarding emotional stress, and encouragement towards correct diet, and relaxation and meditation exercises, will help to minimize the effect of stress, and provide a comprehensive, non-drug approach, to this universal problem.

10. Posture and Correct Body Use

Mechanical stress and dysfunction, · affecting the musculo-skeletal system can often be traced to habitual mis-use of the body. Other causes, including congenital faults, such as supernumary vertebrae, cervical ribs, congenital short leg etc, or traumatic events such as whiplash injuries, or blows and falls, or the effects of long standing emotional stress (see previous chapter), should also be considered.

The daily habits of posture and use, at work and leisure, are frequently the unobtrusive, non-violent, yet persistent factors which mitigate towards somatic dysfunction and the consequences of general ill-health. Posture represents the sum of the mechanical efficiency of the body. It may be read as a book, to assess the integrity, potential, and to some extent, the history of the individual.

The ideal posture is one in which the different segments of the body, the head, neck chest and abdomen are balanced vertically one upon the other so that the weight is borne mainly by the bony framework with a minimum of effort and strain on muscles and ligaments. For such posture to be maintained, special postural muscles must be in a state of constant activity. These have a special physiological property called 'postural activity'. Correct posture is one in which the head is centered over the pelvis the face directed forwards, and the shoulder girdle approximately on the same plane as the pelvis.

The position of the bony framework is determined by the soft tissues which invest, support, bind and move it. Faulty tensions in these soft tissues will lead to abnormalities in the skeletal structures, and therefore to function itself. This may also result in changes in the organs and functions (circulation) which are supported by soft tissues. Not only are the soft tissues subject to gravitational stress, but also to a battery of postural and occupational stresses overlaid with the normal contraction that come with age.

Goldthwait[1] points to the importance of posture in the maintenance of health:

> It has been shown that the main factors which determine the maintenance of the abdominal viscera in position are the diaphragm and abdominal muscles, both of which are relaxed and cease to support in faulty posture. The disturbances in circulation from a low diaphragm and ptosis (sagging organs) may give rise to chronic passive congestion on one or all of the organs of the abdomen and pelvis, since the local as well as general venous drainage may be impeded by the failure of the diaphragmatic pump to do its full work in the drooped body. Furthermore, the drag of these congested organs on their nerve supply, as well as the pressure on the sympathetic ganglia and plexuses (nerve centres), probably causes many irregularities in their function, varying from partial paralysis to overstimulation. Faulty body mechanics in early life, then, become a vital factor in the production of the vicious cycle of chronic diseases and present the chief point of attack in its prevention . . . . In this upright position, as one becomes older, the tendency is for the abdomen to relax and sag more and more, allowing a ptosic condition of the abdominal and pelvic organs unless the supporting lower abdominal muscles are taught to contract properly. As the abdomen relaxes, there is a great tendency to a drooped chest, with a narrowed rib angle, forward shoulders, prominent shoulder blades, a forward position of the head, and probably pronated feet. When the human machine is out of balance, physiological function cannot be perfect; muscles and ligaments are in an abnormal state of tension and strain. A well poised body means a machine working perfectly, with the least amount of muscular effort, and therefore better health and strength in daily life.

Thus an orthodox medical scientist reiterated the osteopathic message. Soft tissues which have been subjected to stresses, of a postural nature, may become chronically stretched or shortened. Normalization, where possible, must involve treatment (soft tissues and joint manipulation), exercise, and above all re-education, to prevent recurrence. A combination of osteopathy and a system of postural re-education, such as Alexander technique, would seem to be the ideal.

Repetitive Stress

Modern man constantly abuses his body. Consider the

compound effects of repetitive industrial or clerical occupations; of driving; of accommodating the body to ill-designed, mass produced furniture or equipment; of physiologically damaging footwear, such as shoes with high heels; and of restrictive undergarments; of habits such as cross-legged sitting, or standing with the weight on only one leg, etc. Just for a moment consider what the body has to cope with in a 'normal day'. Having slept on a too soft bed, the body is obliged to bend or stretch itself through the rigours of washing, shaving and dressing. Wash basins being of uniform size and bodies growing to random lengths can cause stress, even in the simple act of washing the face. The body next finds itself seated in a car, a train or a bus, and then subjected to hours of repetitive duties, either at a desk, at a workbench or in the home, etc. All this is being done on high heels or at a too low or too high desk, or in a seat too deep or too shallow, and in an habitually one-sided manner, with a slouch or stoop. It is not surprising that man has been described as 'a biped animal with backache'.

With this constant repetitive stress we can see why the degeneration of the spinal joints is well advanced by middle-age and why backache, stiff necks and general signs of 'wear and tear' are the rule rather than the exception.

When standing correctly the weight of the body is evenly distributed. A line drawn downwards from the ear should run through the centre of the ankle bone. If it falls in front of this point then the muscles of the neck and spine will be under stress in order to support the head. As the head is held forward of its correct position there occur compensating changes in the normal curves of the spine. These changes, if prolonged, produce permanent alterations which will have their effect on every aspect of body mechanics. Similar problems occur if the head is held to one side or if the pelvis is in a position of forward or backward tilting. The problem is to know how to correct these habitual postural mistakes.

It is interesting to realize that the position of the head and neck in relation to the trunk has a determining effect on the whole economy of the body. The position of the organs of the body is maintained by the fascial bands that support them. The fascia that decides the relative position of the heart, the liver or the spleen, for example, is attached directly to the fascia of the neck, which is joined to the base of the skull. Thus any permanent deviation from normal in this area will have widespread

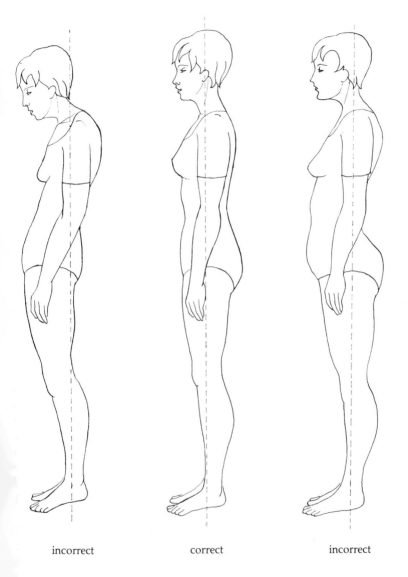

incorrect   correct   incorrect

Two examples of poor posture together with one showing correct
alignment. In the two incorrect examples it can be seen how bad body
mechanics can lead to permanent alteration of muscle tone, organ
displacement and stress on the spinal joints.

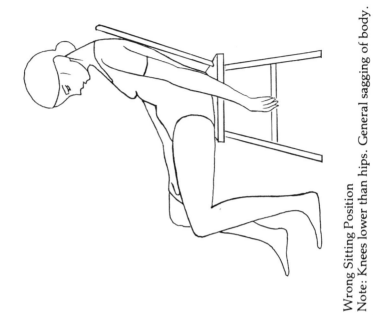

Wrong Sitting Position
Note: Knees lower than hips. General sagging of body.

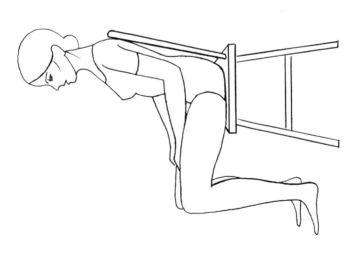

Correct Sitting Position
Note: Knees higher than hips.

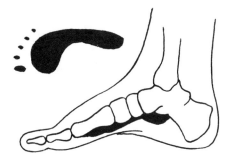

Side view of normal foot.

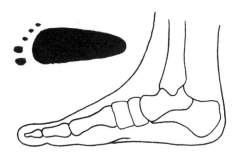

Side view of foot showing dropped arch.

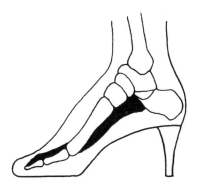

Side view of the effect on the foot of wearing high heels.

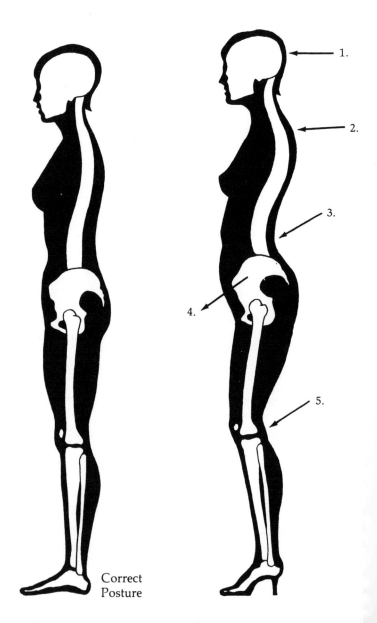

Correct
Posture

The Effect of Wearing High Heels
1. Head forward of its centre of gravity; 2. Thoracic area of spine
rounded; 3. Lumbar area hollowed; 4. Pelvis rotated forward and
abdominal area sagging; 5. Shortening of posterior leg muscles.

ramifications. Once again we see how the body parts inter-relate.

When standing, the crown of the head should be the highest point, not — as is most common — the front of the head. When sitting, the spine should be supported and not allowed to sag. The slope of the upper leg, when sitting, should be from the knee to the hip. That is to say, the knee should be higher than the hip. If this is the case and the buttocks are well back in the chair, the spine will be relaxed and supported. The feet should be so placed that by leaning forward from the sitting position and then straightening the knees, the upright position can be achieved with a minimum of effort. Crosslegged sitting produces twisting strain on the pelvic-lumbar area. It will do no harm for short periods but the danger exists of a habit pattern developing which can help to produce permanent changes in the low-back area.

When walking the head should be held 'tall', not held forward of the centre of gravity of the body. In this way the head becomes less of a heavy weight, which appears to be in danger of falling off its perch on the neck, and more of a 'balloon' floating above the erect body. Think of the graceful movement of a cat or of a ballet dancer; in both examples the head leads and the body appears to follow. Contrast them with the sagging, heavy, round-shouldered appearance so often apparent to any observer. Not only is the appearance so much more pleasing but the effects on general health and energy are demonstrably improved. Bending is essentially produced by the flexion of the knees and hips. A minimum of spinal movement should be required to get down to lift or move an object. If this could be clearly understood and practised there would be a great reduction in spinal problems.

In one-sided, repetitive activities such as digging or sweeping every effort should be made to break the pattern frequently so that other muscles can be used, and those involved in the repetitive movement given a rest.

In one's work it will pay dividends to examine the way simple repetitive activities are performed. For example, I know of a case of severe neck pain which was produced by the habit of holding a telephone receiver between ear and shoulder, thus tilting the head to one side and leaving both hands free. This, when repeated many times a day for some years, resulted in chronic strain.

Ideal Sleeping Position

Sleep should be on a firm surface. The ideal position is to lie on on one side with the head on one medium pillow which is pulled well into the angle between neck and shoulder; thus the head and neck are supported and not allowed to sag or become pushed to one side by too thick a supporting surface. The knees should be flexed so that the lower back is resting in a slightly rounded or neutral position. Sleeping face downwards is undesirable because of the effect on the low back as well as the necessity for the head to be turned to one side.

Physical exercise should involve the use of the whole body; walking, running, cycling and swimming are all desirable. One-sided activities should not be allowed to dominate physical activity to the point of producing imbalance. Exercises of a 'keep fit' nature should be carefully tailored to the individual. Yoga exercises are far more desirable as they are performed in a slow, rhythmic manner rather than in violent, jerky movements so common in the daily dozen!

The way the body is carried in sitting, standing and walking is an ever varying dynamic pattern and the study of this pattern is the study of posture.

The posture of an individual is determined in childhood and the seeds of poor posture in adult life are sown in childhood. Good posture is a rarity — indeed if seen it is instantly recognizable. It is not the stiff military carriage, any more than it is the slouching, sagging posture of the fashion model! One is more likely to recognize good posture in the half naked African tribesman whose graceful carriage enables him to move in an effortless way.

Observe people as they carry out their daily tasks. Few walk well, and one is able to observe a variety of slumped, unhealthy postures when people are sitting. This is an indication of physical weakness, lack of physical exercise, and poor development. It has a direct bearing on health, both physical and mental.

A Common Postural Fault

Lordosis occurs when the pelvis is tilted forward and there is an exaggerated forward curve of the lumbar region of the spine — (high heels, incidentally, throw the pelvis into just this position) There is a corresponding exaggeration of the backward curve o the dorsal spine (kyphosis), and a forward movement of the curve of the neck. These changes of the curves of the spine result in changes in the attached structures, thus throwing strain upon the supporting ligaments, and causing malposition and crowding of the internal organs, circulatory impediments and nerve irritation. The abdominal organs are thrust forward against the wall of the abdomen, the muscles of which become stretched under the constant pressure. The intestines and other supported structures sag and assume a lower position in the abdominal cavity. The liver may rotate forward and the common bile duct may become stretched, in some cases causing interference with bile flow. The pelvic organs are also involved, leading to many of the complications which these days seem to affect women of all ages. There is a sagging of the ovaries, the uterus is tilted forwards and down, with the weight of the abdominal organs resting on it. Varicose veins of the lower bowel (haemorrhoids), and impairment of the reproductive system may result.

With the corresponding crowding of the rib cage there is a decrease in the diameter of the chest. The diaphragm is lowered, leaving the heart in a sagging position, unsupported from below. Both respiratory function and heart action are bound to be less efficient as a result.

Osteopathy can do much to correct the damage — by relaxing tense and congested muscles and joints, by mobilizing the partially immobile joint and by improving general muscle tone. But in order to overcome poor posture permanently there is only one course of action which must be obvious to any intelligent person.

Corrective exercises must firstly overcome the old habits of poor posture and secondly there must be the cultivation and establishment of new habits of good posture. The patient must do much more than exercise — he must consciously assume and maintain correct posture for long, and ever lengthening periods, until correct posture becomes a habit.

The first obstacle to overcome is that of making the individual aware of his tension (or posture). This must be accomplished before he can begin to do anything about it. So, ideally, in postural re-education an instructor is needed in the initial stages, in order to position the body so that the patient can become aware of what it feels like to be in the right position. At first this will feel wrong and it is not until the patient can realize that what feels right is not necessarily right, that progress can begin.

In the long run posture can only be corrected by the individual learning afresh how to use his body machines correctly. The breaking of old habits and the learning of new ones is not easy, but the employment of osteopathy to normalize the soft tissues and joints, will increase the individual's awareness of his body structures, whilst at the same time removing restrictions which can often physically prevent correct use of parts of the body. If one part malfunctions then the whole will, to some extent, malfunction. By breaking into the web of interconnecting factors, with skilled manipulative methods, many complex problems can be resolved.

---

[1] 'Essentials of Body Mechanics' Goldthwait et al.

11. Cranial Osteopathy

One of the greatest pieces of physiological research in the twentieth century was undertaken by William Garner Sutherland D.O. He was one of the early graduates of the original American School of Osteopathy at Kirksville, Missouri in 1900. Whilst a student he noticed that the structure of certain cranial bones, particularly where they joined each other, were bevelled in a striking manner. He noted that there was a marked internal bevel where the squama of the temporal bone overlaps the great wing of the sphenoid and the inferior border of the parietal, which itself displayed a marked external bevel. As he was studying under Dr Still, Sutherland was very conscious of the relationship between structure and function. If these bones were so structured, then, he reasoned, there must be a physiological function related to it. Further investigation of the bones of the skull led him to note many other articulations, such as the 'tongue and groove' junction between the lateral part of the basilar portion of the occiput, where it fits into the medial aspect of the anterior third of the petrous portion of the temporal bone.

Sutherland reasoned that these joints could only make sense if they contributed towards motion between the bones. Against all the accepted medical thinking he reasoned, studied and observed the cranial structures and their functions, with a view to establishing what these were. Gradually, over many years he came to understand the inter-relationship between the bony structures of the cranium and its contents and functions. These include not only the nerve and brain tissues but strong fibrous bands which divide and support the various areas of the brain and which are intimately involved in the motion of the cranial structures. The two main tension membranes are the *Falx*

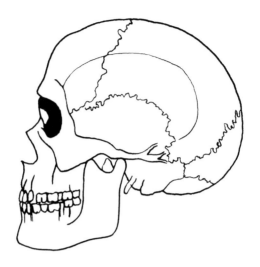

Side view of Adult Cranium.

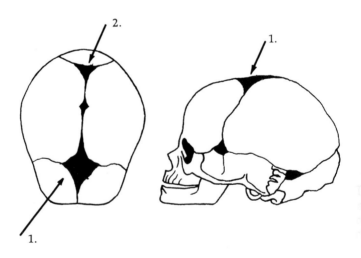

Infant Cranium
Showing: 1. Anterior Fontanelle; 2. Posterior Fontanelle.

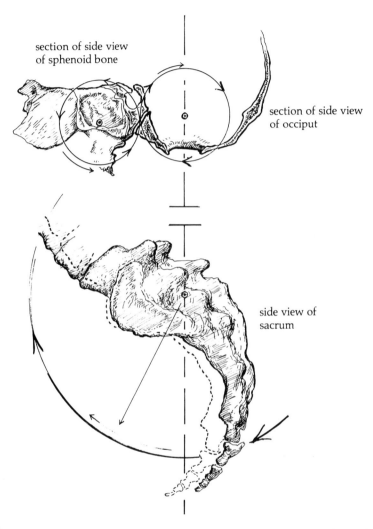

section of side view
of sphenoid bone

section of side view
of occiput

side view of
sacrum

The arrows indicate directions of synchronous co-ordinated alterations in position of the main components of the cranio-sacral mechanism, during flexion (inhalation). The reverse, a return to a neutral position, occurs during extension (exhalation). The dotted line indicates the sacral position at the limit of flexion (inhalation),

Illustration shows cranial and sacral movement during inhalation and exhalation

Cerebri and the *Tentorium Cerebeli.*

The erroneous belief that the skull is a rigid bony structure, and that the sutures are immovable arose from anatomists studying these structures from dried specimens. The study of living bones is quite different. It is a simple matter to feel the resilience of the skull in the living skull, even into adult life.

The bones that make up the skull are, in health, movable and do in fact, move in a rhythmic manner throughout life. The range of this movement is small, but to the trained hand, easily felt. Since nothing in the body is without purpose, this function is reasoned as contributing to the normal running of the body. It might be argued that what is felt is no more than a resiliency, a plasticity, which would be necessary. to avoid the skull being over rigid, and thus in danger of fracturing in case of a blow. This is partly true, but does not explain the rhythmic expansion and contraction that takes place in the skull, independent of the normal respiration and heart beat.

Primary Respiratory Mechanism

Research over the past half century has demonstrated that this movement is part of a mechanism which has been named the 'primary respiratory mechanism'. This involves not only the skull bones, and their contents but, by virtue of strong fibrous tissue connections, the spinal column and the sacrum (the triangular bony structure at the base of the spine). As these structures move (much as the diaphragm and chest move in breathing, but on a much smaller scale) an important circulatory function is being carried out in the skull and throughout the body. Blood and cerebro-spinal fluid are pumped through the intricate channels surrounding the structures of the brain and the central nervous system.

It has been shown under the electron-microscope that the tissue which binds all other tissues together, the connective tissue, or fascia, of the body, has a tubular structure. The cerebro-spinal fluid permeates these structures and carries with it hormonal secretions vital to the health of the body. The most important glands in the body lie within the skull, and their ability to function is now known to be influenced by the efficiency, or otherwise, of the primary respiratory mechanism.

What does all this mean in terms of health and disease? It explains a good deal that was previously unexplained, and opens up the possibility of treating conditions that have proved

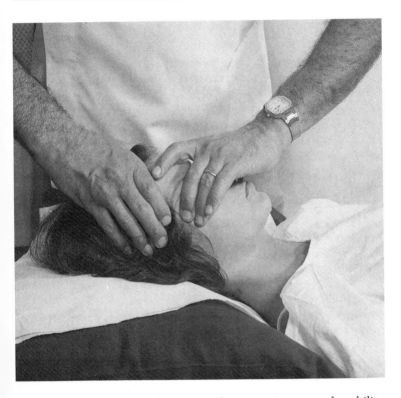

Illustrates cranial manipulation aimed at restoring normal mobility betweeen the zygomatic and the temporal bones. This treatment is extremely gentle. No force is used, only a holding of the appropriate bones whilst the patient's respiratory effort creates the corrective force.

untreatable or stubbornly resistant to treatment, by more conventional methods.

If in adult life there occur blows to the head, whiplash injuries to the neck, heavy dental extractions, blows to the base of the spine, even more subtle structural pressures resulting from new dentures, then the complex mechanism, described above, can be interfered with and a variety of symptoms, local and distant can occur. Local conditions that commonly result from this type of cause include tinnitus (ringing in the ears), Ménière's disease (loss of balance), facial neuralgia, migraine and other headaches, visual disturbances, jaw dysfunction (difficulty in chewing or in opening the mouth) etc. Distant effects can include any sudden changes in the metabolism of the body which could have hormonal origins.

Treatment of Cranial Distortion in New-born Babies

A vast range of conditions have been helped by cranial osteopathy's ability to positively influence the hormonal balance. Such conditions as rheumatoid arthritis, multiple sclerosis, fluid retention, asthma and other allergic problems have all been favourably (together with other natural methods) influenced. The most exciting and important application of this approach is, however, in the treatment of babies and children who have suffered cranial distortion before, during, or soon after birth.

A variety of factors can affect the soft bones and cartilaginous structures of the foetus before, and during birth, and of the infant, soon after. If the mother-to-be has a spinal curve or an acute lumbar curve (hollow back) then the developing foetus may lie in such a way as to crowd or warp, the skull bones. If labour is induced, and the mother's birth canal has not had the opportunity to soften and prepare for the engagement of the foetal head, or if the birth is too rapid and the contractive forces acting on the foetal head are too powerful, or if the process of labour is too long and difficult, the effect on the soft head bones and their supporting structures (tension membranes etc.) can be to so mould them that a return to normal never takes place. If instrument delivery is clumsy this too can cause cranial distortion, and long term problems. This is not to say that forceps delivery is always harmful, indeed it often prevents even worse damage, but it certainly can cause damage, wrongly applied.

If a baby is born prematurely, and is laid on a normal surface then the very weight of the head can have a compressing and warping effect. After all, the foetus has been cushioned in fluid, and a water bed would be a better start as a surface on which to lie, for such a newcomer.

If a newborn child cries too much, refuses food, is stiff and difficult to handle, has sleeping problems, has swallowing difficulty or even shows a distinct preference to lie on one side or not to lie on its back, or is dopey and just 'too good', taking no interest in anything, or rubs or bangs its head, or fails to develop normally, then chances are that there is a cranial distortion. All such children should be seen as soon as possible by a cranial osteopath, as should all cases of cerebral palsy and spasticity.

The treatment methods are exceedingly gentle, and treatment can be started within hours of birth. There is no heroic pushing and pulling which so many people associate with conventional osteopathy, but a gentle, subtle attempt to restore structural normality and with it functional normality (health). Learning the specialized techniques of cranial osteopathy requires lengthy and diligent study and practice. The anatomy and physiology of the skull, and its relationship with other spinal and body structures and functions, is a demanding study. Sensitive and subtle manual skills are required in the application of cranial manipulation, which is not so much concerned with altering the position of bones as with releasing articular strains between the structures and restoring physiological motion. As has been stated, it is in infants and the new-born that the greatest good can be achieved. The following quotation from *The Selected Writings of Beryl Arbuckle D.O.* published in the USA by The National Osteopathic Institute and Cerebral Palsy Foundation (1977) illustrates this:

> The under-developed cerebro-spinal system of the newborn is housed by an immature cranium and vertebral canal. To the skull, with all its intricate construction, so often taken for granted, its physiological movement, little considered and less understood, is attributed the function of protecting the brain. The infant skull is very immature having little ossification and many of the bones are in separate parts, cartilaginous and membranous. The vault consists of very thin bones with but one layer and no bony sutures. The overriding thus possible during delivery is one of nature's provisions for the reduction of cranial size to better enable the passage of the head through the birth canal. If, by chance, for any one of a hundred reasons, that infant is unable to reduce to the full extent this natural moulding it is impossible to prognosticate the severity of the symptoms which may be manifested in later life on account of the persistent unnatural strain throughout the stress bands of the dural membranes. 'An osteopath sees cause in a slight anatomical deviation for the beginning of disease' (A. T. Still). There may result severe or slight muscular handicaps, mental difficulties, from idiocy to mere confusion or general slowness, inability or instability.
>
> The physician who is able to recognize these deviations and able to make the necessary corrections intelligently at the very first sign of slight difficulty, often years before serious symptoms could be manifested, while the child is still in the developing or growing stage, will turn the trouble of today into the triumph of tomorrow.

Glossary of Terms

The following is a selection of definitions taken from a Glossary of Osteopathic Terminology published by the Educational Council on Osteopathic Principles, an organization run by the osteopathic profession in the U.S.A.

Articular strain. The result of forces acting on a joint beyond its capacity to adapt. Refers to stretching of joint components beyond physiological limits, causing damage.

Articulation. (1) The place of union or junction between two or more bones of the skeleton. (2) The active or passive process of moving a joint through its entire range of motion.

Asymmetry. Lack or absence of symmetry of position or motion. Dissimilarity in corresponding parts or organs on opposite sides of the body which are normally alike. Of particular use when describing position or motion alteration resulting from somatic dysfunction.

Barrier (Motion barrier). Limit of unimpeded motion. Anatomic barrier: the limit of motion imposed by anatomic structures. Physiological barrier: functional limits within the anatomic range of motion. Soft tissue tension accumulation which limits the voluntary motion of an articulation. Further motion towards the anatomic barrier can still be induced passively. Pathological barrier: a functional limit within the anatomic range of motion which abnormally diminishes the normal physiological range. May be associated with somatic dysfunction.

Cranial concept. An idea discovered, investigated and developed by W. G. Sutherland D. O. applying osteopathic principles to the skull. It relates the anatomical and physiological mechanisms of the skull that are purported to

represent the action of the primary respiratory mechanism as
the motivating force relevant to the cranio-sacral mechanism
expressed through the cranial rhythmic impulse. The cranial
concept represents the application of the concept of somatic
dysfunction to the cranio-sacral mechanism. Study of the
diagnosis and management of somatic dysfunction as
extended to the cranio-sacral mechanism embraces (1)
introduction and maintenance of somatic dysfunction (2) the
pathological effects of somatic dysfunction (3) specific
methods for palpatory diagnosis and manipulative therapy.

Cranio-sacral mechanism. A term used by Sutherland to
describe the synchronous movement of the sacral base with
the cranial base. This synchrony is accomplished by the
attachment of the dural tube to the foramen magnum and
sacral canal, and probably aided by the cerebro-spinal fluid
fluctuation. It is thought that the foramen magnum moves
forward during flexion of the spheno-basilar articulation
which through the dural tube pulls the sacral base superior
and posterior around a transverse axis at the articular
processes posterior to the canal and through the second sacral
segment.

Facilitation. (1) An increase in afferent stimuli so that the
synaptic threshold is more easily reached; thus there is an
increase in the efficacy of subsequent impulses in that
pathway or synapse. The consequences of increased efficacy
is that continued stimulation produces hyperactive
responses. (2) A clinical concept used by osteopathic
physicians to describe neuro-physiological mechanisms that
create or are created by somatic dysfunction. Most often used
to describe enhancement or reinforcement of neuronal
activity due to increased or abnormal afferent input to a
segment or segments. Increased activity is often triggered
and/or enhanced by adrenergic and sympathetic stimulation.

Inhibition reflex. (1) In osteopathic usage, a term that describes
the application of steady pressure to soft tissues to effect
relaxation and normalize reflex activity. (2) Effect on
antagonist muscles due to reciprocal innervation when the
agonist is stimulated.

Osteopathic lesion. Disturbance in musculo-skeletal structure
and/or function as well as accompanying disturbances of
other biological mechanisms. A term used to describe local
stress or trauma and subsequent effects on other biological

systems (e.g. effects mediated through reflex nerve pathways including autonomic supply to segmentally related organs.)

Osteopathic manipulative therapy. Any of several manual methods used to alleviate painful and distressing symptoms of disease or injury by creating mechanical displacement of fluids, soft tissues, or bony structures. Purported to facilitate removal of toxic materials and induce neuro-vascular and neuro-muscular effects.

Osteopathy. A system of health care founded by Andrew Taylor Still (1828-1917) and based on the theory that the body is capable of making its own remedies against disease and other toxic conditions when it is in normal structural relationship and has favourable environmental conditions and adequate nutrition. It utilizes generally accepted physical, pharmacological and surgical methods of diagnosis and therapy, while placing strong emphasis on the importance of body mechanics and manipulative methods to detect and correct faulty structure and function. (Author's note: The reference to pharmacological and surgical methods does not apply to osteopaths in the U.K. — see Chapter 3.)

Physiological motion of the spine. Descriptive of spinal motion proposed by Harrison H. Fryette D.O. The three major principles are (1) when the spine is in a neutral position (easy normal) and sidebending is introduced, the bodies of the vertebrae will rotate towards the convexity; (2) when the spine is either forward or backward bent and sidebending is introduced, the vertebrae will rotate towards the concavity; (3) initiating motion of a vertebral segment in any plane of motion will modify the movement of that segment in the other planes of motion.

Primary machinery of life. The neuro-musculo-skeletal system. A term used by I. M. Korr Ph.D. to denote that body parts act together to transmit and modify force and motion through which man acts out life. It receives its direction from the central nervous system acting in response to continued sensory input from the internal and external environment.

Primary respiratory mechanism. In cranio-sacral terminology, a term used to describe the interdependent function of several anatomical and physiological components of the central nervous system. This primary respiratory function is purported to have remote effects on the entire body. Usually refers specifically to the inherent pulsating movement of the brain and spinal cord (8-12 cycles per minute); a rhythmic fluctuation of the cerebro-spinal fluid and circulation independent of pulmonary respiration and heart rate; the articular mobility of the cranial bones; and the involuntary movement of the sacrum between the ilia seemingly correlated and interdependent with the rhythmic cerebrospinal fluid fluctuations.

Reflex. An involuntary nervous system response to a sensory input. The sum total of any particular involuntary activity. Conditioned reflex: one that does not occur naturally in the organism or system, but that may be developed by regular association of some physiological function with an unrelated outside event. So the physiological function starts whenever the outside event occurs. Red reflex: the erythematous reaction of the skin in an area that has been mildly stimulated mechanically (e.g. by palpatory examination.) The reflex is greater in degree and duration in an area of acute somatic dysfunction. Somato-somatic reflex: localized somatic stimuli producing patterns of reflex response in segmentally related somatic structures. Somato-visceral reflex: localized somatic stimulation producing patterns of reflex response in segmentally related visceral structures. Viscero-somatic reflex: localized visceral stimuli producing patterns of reflex response in segmentally related somatic structures. Viscero-visceral reflex: localized visceral stimuli producing patterns of reflex response in segmentally related visceral structures. Also called viscero-somato-visceral reflex.

Somatic dysfunction. Impaired or altered function of related components of the somatic (body framework) system — skeletal, arthrodial and myofascial structures, and related vascular, lymphatic and neural elements. The positional and motion aspects of somatic dysfunction may be described using three parameters: (1) The position of the element as determined by palpation; (2) the direction in which motion is freer; (3) the direction in which motion is restricted. Acute and chronic somatic dysfunction are identified by A.R.T. (Asymmetry, Restriction of motion and Tenderness.)

Tissue texture abnormality. Any palpable change in tissues from skin to periaticular structures that represents any combination of the following signs: vasodilitation oedema, flaccidity, contraction, contracture, fibrosis, and the following symptoms: itching, pain, tenderness, paresthesias.

Types of TTA include: bogginess, thickening, stringiness, ropiness, firmness or hardening, increased or decreased temperature, increased or decreased moisture

Trigger point (myofascial). A small hypersensitive site that, when stimulated, consistently produces a reflex mechanism that gives rise to referred pain or other manifestations. The response is specific, in a constant reference zone and consistent from person to person.

Bibliography

Arbuckle, Beryl, *The Selected Writings of Beryl Arbuckle D.O.* National Osteopathic Institute and Cerebral Palsy Foundation (U.S.A.).

Brookes, Denis, *Lectures on Cranial Osteopathy.* Thorsons.

Chaitow, Leon, *Neuro-Muscular Technique.* Thorsons.

Fryett, Harrison H., *Principles of Osteopathic Technique.* American Academy of Osteopathy.

Gelb, Harold and others, *Clinical Management of Head, Neck and T.M.J. Pain and Dysfunction.* W.B. Saunders and Co.

Hoag, J. M., W. V. Cole, S. G. Bradford, *Osteopathic Medicine.* McGraw-Hill.

Korr, Irvin M., *The Collected Papers of Irvin M. Korr.* American Academy of Osteopathy.

——, *The Neurobiological Mechanisms in Manipulative Therapy*, Plenum Press, New York.

Magoun, Harold, Osteopathy in the Cranial Field. Sutherland Cranial Teaching Foundation.

Northup, George W., *Osteopathic Medicine: an American Reformation.* American Osteopathic Association.

Still, Andrew T., *Philosophy of Osteopathy.* American Academy of Osteopathy.

Stoddard, Alan, *Manual of Osteopathic Technique.* Hutchinson.

——, *Manual of Osteopathic Practice.* Hutchinson.

Yearbooks of the Academy of Applied Osteopathy.

Colleges of Osteopathy in the U.K.

The British College of Naturopathy and Osteopathy
6 Netherhall Gardens, London NW3 5RR
(Tel: 01-435 7830)

The British School of Osteopathy
16 Buckingham Gate, London SW1E 6LB
(Tel: 01-828 9479)

The European School of Osteopathy
104 Tonbridge Road, Maidstone, Kent
(Tel: 0622 671558)

The London College of Osteopathy
8 Boston Place, London NW2
(Tel: 01-262 1128)
The College of Osteopaths Educational Trust
21 Manor Road North, Wallington Surrey SM6 7NS
(Tel: 01-647 2452)

Index